PRACTISING PREVENTION

PRACTISING PREVENTION

Articles published in
the *British Medical Journal*

Published by the British Medical Association
Tavistock Square, London WC1H 9JR

ISBN 0 7279 0155 9

Made and printed in England by
The Devonshire Press
Barton Road, Torquay

Preface

by the Editor

British Medical Journal

Prevention is a word on everybody's lips these days, but how exactly can general practitioners find time in their busy surgeries to start preventive activities? For it is to general practitioners and their teams that we must look for the huge increase in preventive activity that we need: no other institution can cope. In a practical and authoritative way this book tells general practitioners of all the preventive activities that they might undertake. Nevertheless, the authors, most of whom are themselves general practitioners, recognise that a doctor cannot spend all his working life preventing disease, and they spell out which activities will produce the richest rewards. They also explain how many of the activities can be undertaken by other members of the practice team.

No matter what kind of practices doctors work in they will be able to extract from this book practical preventive programmes that will suit them. And there is a great deal to be achieved: research has shown that general practitioners are more effective than anybody in, for instance, helping people to stop smoking. Simple advice from general practitioners resulted in 5% of smokers stopping, which means 25 smokers for the average general practitioner and half a million people for the whole of Britain. The saving in mortality and morbidity is immense, and there is every reason to suppose that general practitioners can be equally effective in other preventive activities.

STEPHEN LOCK
1983

Contents

vii

Contents

Prevention—what does it mean?

GODFREY FOWLER

The traditional view of the doctor's role is changing. Managing symptoms is no longer adequate and the scope for doctors—particularly general practitioners—to influence the health of their patients by preventive medicine is being acknowledged more and more. General practice provides a good framework for preventive medicine. Virtually everyone in Britain is registered with a general practitioner and, more importantly for prevention, each general practitioner has a defined list of patients. Two thirds of these patients consult him at least once a year and nearly all of them at least once every five years. Every day almost one million consultations take place in general practice in this country. The fact that much disease is "below the surface" is illustrated by the diagram of the "iceberg of disease."[1]

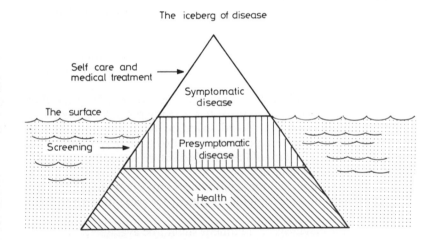

The iceberg of disease

PRIMARY, SECONDARY, AND TERTIARY PREVENTION

The ideal form of prevention is removing the cause—so called *primary* prevention. Much illness today is due not to external agents but to unhealthy human behaviour. Diseases related to smoking are an obvious example, and avoiding cigarette smoking is the most important form of primary prevention. It requires the doctor to add an educational role to his diagnostic and therapeutic ones. *Secondary* prevention is the early detection of disease before symptoms, or

Prevention—what does it mean?

disordered function, appear and when action may stop or even reverse the disease process. Detecting hypertension is an example. In secondary prevention *risk factors* are acknowledged, and their presence is associated with an increased chance of developing a disease. Raised blood pressure and smoking are risk factors, both being associated with the development of cardiovascular disease and smoking with respiratory and other diseases. Risk factors may be asymptomatic—until the damage is done. *Tertiary* prevention is the management of established disease to avoid or limit the development of a disability or handicap. Supervision of diabetic patients is an example of tertiary prevention.

SCREENING

Screening is synonymous with secondary prevention. Screening is the scrutiny of a population to find those who have risk factors for a disease or have the disease itself. Case finding is a form of screening in which the initiative is limited to the opportunistic approach: the patient seeking advice from the doctor about symptoms is at the same time questioned, examined, or investigated for an unrelated condition. This contrasts with the more aggressive pursuit of the individual with no complaints to which a narrow definition of screening may sometimes be confined and which is a feature of population surveys. The term "anticipatory care" has also been used to describe case finding.

Two views prevail about screening. The evangelists argue that doctors should be more committed to screening procedures than they are. The cynics, on the other hand, maintain that few of the screening procedures that have been properly evaluated have been shown to be valid. The criteria that should be satisfied before screening is adopted have been listed by Wilson[2]:
—the condition screened for should be an important one;
—there should be an acceptable treatment for patients with the disease;
—facilities for diagnosis or treatment should be available;
—there should be a recognised latent or early symptomatic stage;
—there should be a suitable test or examination;
—the test or examination should be acceptable to the population;
—the natural history of the condition, including the development from a latent to a declared disease, should be adequately understood;
—there should be an agreed policy on whom to treat as patients;
—the cost of case finding (including diagnosis and subsequent treatment of patients) should be economically balanced in relation to civil expenditure on medical care as a whole;
—case finding should be a continuous and not a once for all project.

Prevention—what does it mean?

ETHICAL CONSIDERATIONS

Screening and case finding impose obligations on the doctor over and above those to which he is normally subject. In the conventional consultation concerned with illness the patient seeks the doctor's help, and though the doctor accepts the obligation to try to fulfil the patient's needs, there is no commitment to success. In screening or case finding, on the other hand, it is the doctor who takes the initiative and thus implies that his intervention.will benefit the patient. There is a presumption not only that the abnormality that is sought will, if present, be detected, but that detection will lead to effective treatment. Moreover, there may be costs to the patient—anxiety, inconvenience, possible discomfort, and even potential harm.

A further complication is false positive and false negative results. A false positive result indicates that there is an abnormality when there is not; while a false negative result is the failure to identify the abnormality when it is in fact present. While a false positive result will cause unnecessary distress to the person and maybe expose him to the hazards of treatment that is also unnecessary, a false negative result will be followed by erroneous reassurance and failure to treat the abnormality which in fact exists.

HEALTH EDUCATION

Preventive medicine in the nineteenth century was based largely on changes in the environment. Because much disease in the twentieth century is caused by the unhealthy habits of individuals, modern prevention depends on achieving changes in human behaviour. Smoking, overeating, alcohol abuse, lack of exercise, and accidents are major contributors to morbidity and mortality. Health education is the first step in achieving healthy behaviour. Cynics may dispute the effectiveness of health education in producing healthy behaviour, but there is accumulating evidence of such effectiveness.[3] General practitioners may also be reluctant to see themselves as health educators but should remind themselves that the word "doctor" means teacher and that "of all the many and varied sources of health information available to the adult population it is the general practitioner who is the most trusted and whose advice has most impact."[4]

ROLE OF THE GENERAL PRACTITIONER

There can be little doubt that if preventive medicine is worth while general practice provides important opportunities to practise it. The general practitioner and his team are available and accessible to most of the population. Most important, they have contact with people who are least likely to seek preventive help themselves, yet whose needs are the greatest. The credibility of a general practitioner's advice is high

Prevention—what does it mean?

and the role of health educator therefore all the more important. Continuity of care—the continuing relationship between the general practitioner and the patient—is as important to preventive medicine as it is to therapeutic medicine.

REFERENCES

[1] Last JM. The iceberg: completing the clinical picture in general practice. *Lancet* 1963; ii:28–31.
[2] Wilson JMG. In: Teeling Smith J, ed. *Surveillance and early diagnosis in general practice: proceedings of colloquium.* London: Office of Health Economics, 1966: 5–10.
[3] Russell MAH, Wilson C, Taylor C, Baker CD. Effect of general practitioners' advice against smoking. *Br Med J* 1979;ii:231–5.
[4] McCron R, Budd J. Communication and health education. Prepared for Health Education Council. University of Leicester Centre for Mass Communication Research, October 1979: Chapter 8, unpublished.

What is preventable?

GODFREY FOWLER

"Prevention is better than cure." But it is one thing to know the cause and another to remove or modify it—and yet another, by doing so, to prevent the disease. One difficulty is that there are many uncertainties about the effectiveness of various preventive measures. Not that this is peculiar to preventive medicine: few aspects of therapeutic medicine have been shown to be of undoubted benefit when rigorously appraised. General practitioners are used to having to act on less than adequate information, and there is evidence that some important preventive activities are effective.

The general practitioner is particularly well placed to practise preventive medicine because he has ready access to a defined population, is in frequent contact with those most in need, can identify those at particular risk, will be concerned with the management of any problems detected, and can combine prevention with cure and care. Most importantly, opportunities for intervention arise during normal care when the patient has sought medical help, albeit for an unrelated problem.

IMMUNISATION

Immunisation against infectious diseases is one form of primary prevention, the value of which is undisputed. For most doctors diphtheria is a disease of historical interest only, but many will have personal knowledge of the effects of others such as polio and measles before effective immunisation was introduced. More recently the resurgence of whooping cough after the decline in pertussis immunisation has been a reminder of the importance of this form of prevention. Moreover, despite the availability of safe, reliable vaccines, there are still about 100 cases of tetanus (with its high fatality rate) each year and several hundred babies born with congenital malformations due to rubella.

CONTRACEPTION

Contraception is another important aspect of primary prevention and one in which general practitioners have played a greater part in recent years—95% now provide family planning services. Despite this, more than 100 000 pregnancies are terminated each year, indicating that there is considerable scope for promoting contraceptive practice.

PREGNANCY AND CHILDHOOD

Other preventive activities that have been incorporated into the

5

What is preventable?

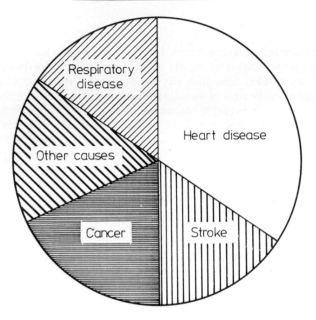

routine work of many practices for some considerable time are antenatal care and paediatric surveillance. Antenatal care was the first screening procedure to be widely adopted in general practice. Identifying those women at greater risk of having an abnormal pregnancy or confinement is an important function of antenatal care, and though many of the procedures conducted on pregnant women remain unevaluated the overall benefits of antenatal care are generally accepted. The value of routine screening examinations in childhood is more debatable, though few would dispute the worth of selective ones.

CANCER OF CERVIX AND BREAST

Although cervical cytology was the first screening procedure to be introduced for the detection of malignant disease its effectiveness has only recently become fully acknowledged. The major problem is implementing screening, particularly applying it to those most at risk of having cancer of the cervix. The case for breast cancer screening is, however, less clearly established. Although this is the commonest malignancy in women, killing about 12 000 every year (more than five times as many as those killed by cervical cancer) and is the commonest

6

cause of death in women aged 25 to 54, scope for its prevention seems limited.

CARDIOVASCULAR DISEASE

But the main cause of death in developed countries is arterial disease—particularly coronary heart disease and strokes. As the figure illustrates, together they account for roughly half of all deaths, and coronary heart disease alone for almost half of all deaths in middle aged men. A recent review said that "about half of all strokes and a quarter of all deaths from coronary heart disease in people under 70 are probably preventable by the application of existing knowledge."

This presents a major challenge for general practitioners, particularly because it requires a shift towards doing more health education. The need for this arises out of the fact that arterial disease—and coronary heart disease in particular—seems to be largely determined by an unhealthy lifestyle and harmful habits. Smoking, overeating, faulty diets, excessive alcohol intake, lack of exercise, and raised blood pressure have been shown with varying degrees of certainty to contribute to cardiovascular disease.

PSYCHIATRIC DISORDERS

Prevention of psychiatric illness has been especially neglected. The importance of psychosocial factors in illness presented to the general practitioner and the high proportion of patients consulting their general practitioner who have psychological illness highlight the potential scope for its prevention. Preventive action at times of life change—such as parenthood, retirement, and bereavement—may avert the development of psychiatric disorders and alcoholism and reduce the risk of self injury and suicide.

CHRONIC DISEASE

Finally, there are opportunities in general practice for tertiary prevention—managing established disease so as to prevent or limit disability or handicap. The careful supervision of patients known to have diabetes, hypertension, and other chronic diseases is preventive medicine in a form which is perhaps more readily identified with the therapeutic role of the doctor.

COMPLIANCE

All these aspects of preventive medicine require not only action by doctors—be it advice or "clinical" action—but also cooperation or "compliance" by patients. In case it should be thought that this problem is peculiar to prevention we should remember that the fate of

7

What is preventable?

the medication we prescribe may be at least as uncertain as that of our advice.

FURTHER READING

Health and prevention in primary care. Report from General Practice No. 18. London: Royal College of General Practitioners, 1981.

Prevention of arterial disease in general practice. Report from General Practice No. 19. London: Royal College of General Practitioners, 1981.

Prevention of psychiatric disorders in general practice. Report from General Practice No. 20. London: Royal College of General Practitioners, 1981.

Family planning: an exercise in preventive medicine. Report from General Practice No. 21. London: Royal College of General Practitioners, 1981.

Opportunities for prevention: the consultation

S A SMAIL

Since the inception of the National Health Service strategies for preventive care in general practice have often centred on establishing special screening programmes or clinics, such as cervical cytology or well baby clinics. Yet many doctors now appreciate the wide potential for preventive care that exists in every consultation. Roughly 75% of patients consult at least once every year,[1] and nearly all patients are seen at least once every five years. Patients not only trust their own doctor's general advice about health but also they expect more explanation and discussion in the consultation.[1] Patients are therefore receptive to advice about prevention during the consultation. Indeed, the "illness interview" may be the only opportunity to discuss prevention with those patients who are unlikely ever to attend special clinics set up to provide preventive or anticipatory care.

PERCEIVING OPPORTUNITIES

The most obvious examples of preventive care are those related to the problem presented by the patient. Doctors feel most comfortable discussing secondary prevention (screening) and tertiary prevention (treatment), though by inclination and training they may still find it easier to reach for the prescription pad rather than discuss preventive action with the patient. Yet patients can only avoid recurrence of problems as diverse as backache, nutritional anaemia, or attacks of gout if they fully understand the cause of the condition and ways to avoid it. Such explanation and advice has been called "patient education;" and its importance in primary care is now widely recognised, particularly in the United States,[2] though it is neglected surprisingly often by British general practitioners.[1] Patients readily accept this type of advice and invariably recognise its relevance.

There are opportunities for preventive care that are quite unrelated to the presenting problem in nearly every consultation.[3] Doctors often feel diffident about discussing primary prevention or health promotion with patients, but nevertheless patients seem to appreciate such advice and there is some evidence that it is effective. It is easy to persuade a patient who has a chest infection or has recently suffered a myocardial infarction to give up smoking, but a surprisingly high success rate may also be achieved by giving the simple advice to stop smoking to all smokers, whether or not they have consulted with a problem related to smoking.[4] Other opportunities might include advice about diet, exercise, or contraception.

Specific screening or case finding procedures may be carried out

9

Opportunities for prevention: the consultation

during consultations. Most general practitioners now agree that patients over 35 years of age should be screened for hypertension during the consultation, but few actually do it.[5] Patients may also be advised about immunisation or cervical cytology—preventive care that has the added advantage of being potentially profitable for the practice. Although immunisation of infants is generally carried out routinely, it is easy to forget that middle aged and elderly patients may never have had a primary course of tetanus toxoid injections.

Perhaps the best opportunities for offering advice are when patients consult for preventive care—for an antenatal visit or for immunisation—when other topics of primary or secondary prevention may easily be introduced. An initial request for contraceptive advice presents a wide range of possibilities and may require discussion of several of the following points:

—attitudes to and knowledge of contraception, conception, and venereal disease;
—smoking (particularly in relation to oral contraception);
—rubella immunity;
—cervical cytology;
—breast self examination;
—diet;
—potential risks of genetic disease.

COMMUNICATING WITH THE PATIENT

The patient is most likely to accept preventive advice if he or she feels that the doctor has fully understood the problem. This is only possible if the doctor has taken the trouble to find out the patient's views and beliefs about health and disease.[6] The patient can then be given advice that is congruent with his or her own beliefs, and there is less risk that the advice will be inappropriate. There are dangers in an overenthusiastic approach to preventive care, particularly if the doctor gives a great deal of heavy handed proscriptive advice. There is some risk of alienating the patient, but this may be avoided by showing sensitivity to the patient's own views. After discussion with the patient it is important for the doctor to check that the patient fully understands what he has said. Although patients obviously need to understand advice before either accepting it or acting on it, in fact it is unusual for doctors to check patients' understanding of advice given.

Thus it is essential to ensure that there is sufficient two way communication in the consultation if preventive advice is to be successful. Many general practitioners think that they possess ample innate skills in communication, but there is evidence that although a large part of the consultation may be spent in "exposition" to the patient[7] much of the communication is one way from doctor to patient

Opportunities for prevention: the consultation

and may leave patients confused.[6] Doctors can, however, improve their skills in communication, particularly by using audio or video recordings of their consultations to provide feedback of their own performance.[8][9] This should improve the effectiveness of any preventive advice given during the consultation.

To reinforce the points made the patient may be given a simple leaflet so that he or she may refer to it later, knowing that the contents carry the doctor's approval. Practices may wish to design their own leaflets[10]—remembering that the language must be kept very simple. But there are now many leaflets specifically designed for use in the consultation—for example, the "Give up Smoking" leaflet available from the Health Education Council.

EXTENDING INITIATIVES TAKEN DURING THE CONSULTATION

Some general practitioners acknowledge the importance of preventive advice but feel that their consultations are inevitably so brief that it is difficult if not impossible to deal with anything other than the presenting problem. Much preventive advice, however, may be given very quickly, and initiatives taken in the consultation may be extended by other practice staff.

All members of the practice team should agree a list of priorities that may be reviewed at intervals. Initial objectives might include advice about smoking and rubella, and flu immunisation. Each member of the practice may then develop his or her own contribution. In the consultation the main task is to identify preventive opportunities. Other staff members may then give further advice or carry out specific procedures—either at the same visit or later. The receptionist can supply appropriate literature and ensure that details of preventive action are entered in the patients' records, and the practice nurse can carry out immunisations, teach breast self examination, or check blood pressures. The health visitor already has a general responsibility for giving preventive advice to patients but also can reinforce specific advice given during the consultation. The most important step, however, is for every member of the practice to develop a sensitivity for preventive opportunities at each and every contact with patients.

REFERENCES

[1] Cartwright A, Anderson R. Patients and their doctors, 1977. Occasional Paper No. 8. London: Royal College of General Practitioners, 1979.
[2] Squyres WD. *Patient education: an enquiry into the state of the art.* New York: Springer, 1980.
[3] Stott NCH, Davis RH. The exceptional potential in each primary care consultation. *J R Coll Gen Pract* 1979;**29**:201–5.
[4] Fleming DM, Lawrence MSTA. An evaluation of recorded information about preventive measures in 38 practices. *J R Coll Gen Pract* 1980;**31**:615–20.

Opportunities for prevention: the consultation

5 Russell MAH, Wilson C, Taylor C, Baker CD. Effect of general practitioners' advice against smoking. *Br Med J* 1979;ii:231–5.
6 Svarstad BL. Physician-patient communication and patient conformity with medical advice. In: Mechanic D, ed. *Growth of bureaucratic medicine.* New York: Wiley & Sons, 1976:220–37.
7 Bartlett EE. Contributions of consumer health education to primary care practice: a review. *Med Care* 1980;**8**:862–71.
8 Walton JN. *Talking with patients: a teaching approach.* London: Nuffield Provincial Hospitals Trust, 1980.
9 Davis RH, Jenkins M, Smail SA, *et al.* Teaching with audiovisual recordings of consultations. *J R Coll Gen Pract* 1980;**30**:333–6.
10 Muir Gray JA. Preparing a leaflet for patient education. *Br Med J* 1982;**284**:1171–2.

Preparing a leaflet for patient education

J A MUIR GRAY

It is now generally accepted that patients can recall only a few facts after a consultation with the general practitioner. Furthermore, the parts of doctors' advice that are remembered are not necessarily the most important, and the patient is often unable to repeat correctly aspects of the advice that he has managed to remember. In the past this frequently was blamed on the patient's stupidity or inattention, but it is now appreciated—albeit not universally—that the fault often lies with the doctor and that by observing certain simple guidelines the amount of information that the patient can retain may be increased. Even with the best technique, however, most patients will not remember all the points that the doctor believes to be most important. One way of increasing the effectiveness of communication is to complement the spoken advice with written material. The most effective medium would be a summary of the advice given in the consultation written specifically for each patient, but this is impossible and a leaflet suitable for all people who have a particular condition or problem has to serve instead.

"Leaflets" have, quite rightly, been widely and fiercely criticised, but a leaflet prepared in accordance with some simple guidelines can effectively contribute to both prevention and treatment if it is used to complement the advice given during a consultation. Indeed, it can be argued that many consultations are unnecessarily ineffective because the doctor relies exclusively on spoken communication. Leaflets have their place in medical practice—and that place is not always the wastepaper basket.

THE MESSAGE

The message in any leaflet written to encourage prevention should always emphasise four points:

(1) The seriousness of the problem. The aim should be to create concern but not overwhelming anxiety—for example, to say that smoking causes lung cancer but not to describe the suffering of a cancer patient in gory detail.

(2) The susceptibility of the reader. The statement that there are 185 000 deaths from coronary heart disease in Britain each year impresses the policy maker or epidemiologist. The individual, however, wants to know whether or not he is susceptible—for example, present him with a list of risk factors for heart disease that he can use to assess his personal level of risk.

(3) The benefits that will result from following the advice. It is

13

Preparing a leaflet for patient education

insufficient to say that high blood pressure increases the risk of a stroke; it is also necessary to state that a reduction in blood pressure is associated with a reduction in risk. If there are any other benefits that will follow from taking the advice—that is, benefits other than reducing the risk of disease—they should be emphasised. For example, say: "If you lose weight you will feel better and fitter and look more attractive;" as well as emphasise the beneficial effects of weight reduction on the metabolic problems of mature onset diabetes.

(4) The difficulties the patient may face. Try to think of the difficulties that the patient may have in following advice, and give specific advice on how these may be minimised.

STYLE OF THE MESSAGE

Having chosen the facts that are to be included, it is essential to set them out clearly. Writing clearly and simply is difficult. It is more difficult than writing long and complicated sentences, with commas and semicolons separating a concatenation of clauses. It takes time and practice to learn how to write simply and clearly, but there are a few guidelines that should be observed:

(1) Don't use too many technical terms. When a term is first used it should always be defined. On the other hand, don't use too few technical terms. It is patronising to use terms like "tummy" when the technical term is in common use.

(2) Use short sentences.

(3) Use large print—capital letters on an ordinary typewriter is a good size of writing for older patients (though not for most of us).

(4) Put the most important information at the beginning and then repeat it towards the end of the text, perhaps as a succinct summary of the advice.

(5) Avoid general vague instructions such as "take more exercise;" or "eat less fat." Be specific and precise. If you do not feel that you can be precise when writing a leaflet or handout leave a blank space in the leaflet for specific instructions tailored to the individual's needs. Never be afraid that you will be too detailed. Nearly always the mistake is to give general exhortations that aggravate anxiety without changing behaviour. Specific, precise instructions reduce anxiety and are more likely to be effective.

The difficulty of writing clearly should not be underestimated. The doctor who wishes to acquire the skill can learn how to draft plain English by reading "the tabloids" with care and attention to style. Try reading the *Daily Mail* or *Express* or the *Sun, Star,* or *Mirror* carefully at least once a week. Study the leader column for plain prose at its clearest, even if you do not agree with the opinions expressed. An even

14

more effective way of learning, however, is to pilot the leaflet and seek criticism.

PREPARING THE MEDIUM

So much for the message, now for the medium. No amount of care in presentation can improve an incomprehensible message, but a clearly written message may be obfuscated by poor presentation. The rules of leaflet preparation may be summarised simply:

(1) Write in short paragraphs. Use headings to break the text into short sections. If listing several facts or points set them in a line and indent them one centimetre to highlight their importance.

(2) Try the question and answer style as one of your drafts. Market research has shown that it is an effective means of keeping the reader's attention.

(3) Leave space for writing in "personalised" advice. For example, you can give a leaflet on exercise and say: "There are two points that are particularly important for you to remember so I am going to write them down here."

(4) Try to find ways in which the reader can use the leaflet to assess his condition or record his progress—self monitoring improves compliance. For example, leave a space for him to write down what he finds most difficult about following the advice so that he can discuss this with the doctor or health visitor when he consults again.

(5) Pilot your leaflet and try to evaluate its comprehensibility. Remember that many patients are reluctant to criticise anything their general practitioner produces honestly because they are reluctant to hurt his feelings. Try to enlist the help of a medical student or student health visitor or one of the administrative staff in the health centre. Remember that the local health authority can dispense small sums from research funds for this type of action research.

The well prepared leaflet is a useful medium for communication which has had a bad press. If prepared by the general practitioner for his own patients it can make an effective contribution.

Making a start

L I ZANDER

The importance of preventive care is being increasingly stressed,[1] but the general practitioner needs to consider carefully how to best use his potential in this field.[2] Improving our level of performance is less an issue of increasing knowledge than of changing our attitudes and the way we work. Although preventive care should not be seen as an activity that is separate or independent from normal practice management, there are certain important differences that should be recognised, as they provide important guidelines on how performance may be improved.

Routine clinical care	*Preventive care*
Care initiated by patient	Care initiated by doctor
Nature of care is usually unpredictable	Nature of care is predictable
Demand for care is immediate	Provision is non-urgent
Focus of attention is the individual patient	Management of "target" groups
Management usually concerns the doctor	Management often provided by non-medical members of the health care team
Good records are helpful	Good information system is absolutely essential
Audit of outcome is highly complex	Audit of care provided is fairly simple

ORGANISING CARE

The doctor's principal clinical activity is conducting the consultation, and the possibilities for undertaking preventive care at this time have been well described by Stott and Davis[3] and Smail.[4] During normal consulting sessions, however, the general practitioner faces the dilemma of conflicting interests, as his principal preoccupation will be to cope with the problems presented to him. If he is to play an effective part in preventive care the practitioner must assume responsibility for deciding both the nature of the care to be provided and how this is to be achieved. The scope of a preventive approach to patient care may be considered under the following headings:

Objectives	*Examples of care*
Prevention of certain diseases	Immunisation programmes
	Cervical cytology screening
Prevention of the complication of certain conditions	Long term management—for example, hypertension
	Long term follow up—for example, postgastrectomy care
Prevention or modification of certain behaviour patterns	Advice about alcohol intake, smoking, diet, etc
Prevention of certain unwanted events	Family planning

16

As the content of much preventive care is predictable, non-urgent, and concerns specific patient groups, this should be reflected in the way that delivery of care is organised.

A TEAM ACTIVITY

The question of how and by whom different types of preventive care are to be undertaken is critical to its success, and relates to factors such as training, motivation, availability, and accessibility. The health visitor and the midwife have already well established roles in well baby care and antenatal supervision, and hypertension, cervical cytology, and rubella immunisation programmes are effectively carried out by trained nursing staff.[5] The role of the nurse and other members of the team in running well women clinics, family planning, and health education programmes can be expanded considerably. The doctor's participation may be minimal, his critical function being to plan and coordinate.

PRACTICE INFORMATION SYSTEM

A satisfactory data system is an absolute prerequisite if an effective programme of prevention is to be practised. The clinical record of each patient should not be considered in isolation but seen rather as the central component of an integrated information system of the total practice population. The system should aim at:

(1) Identifying those factors whose effect on health care may be modified by preventive action.

(2) Identifying risk factors in individuals and in vulnerable groups in the practice population.

(3) Providing data concerning the level of preventive care undertaken.

Individual clinical record

The patient's clinical record should include: (a) certain physical factors amenable to change—for example, weight, blood pressure; (b) certain behavioural characteristics, such as excessive smoking, drinking, or gambling; (c) occupation, identifying particular risks or stresses—for example, publican, miner; (d) family history of conditions with genetic implications; (e) allergies and sensitivities; (f) morbidity record of conditions requiring long term follow up (postgastrectomy patients) or long term management (pernicious anaemia, hypertension); (g) details of what preventive procedures have been undertaken, such as immunisation, contraception (advice given and method used), and cervical cytology.

Making a start

Record of practice population

The age-sex register is the basic tool necessary to practise preventive care in the practice as a whole. It defines the population for whose care the practitioner is responsible and enables him to identify cohorts of vulnerable or target groups for whom specific preventive care is indicated.

A practice morbidity register will allow monitoring of specific chronic conditions and their management, and when linked to the age-sex register will enable specific preventive programmes to be planned. Many different record formats, including summary cards, flow charts, and morbidity registers, have been designed, and the Central Information Service at the Royal College of General Practitioners will provide useful information and advice on how to set up age-sex and morbidity registers.

Computers

Having a microcomputer in the practice can make a major contribution to preventive care by facilitating data collection and retrieval. A more important benefit to be derived from its predicted widespread use[6] is that by synthesising a range of different items of information—such as age, sex, weight, blood pressure, and smoking habits—a level of risk identification is possible that could not be achieved by manual methods.

AUDIT OF CARE

Audit is a necessary stimulus for improvement. Some form of assessment should ideally be part of every programme of preventive care, so that information concerning its delivery is readily available and regularly fed back to those responsible for providing it.

PRACTICE ORGANISATION AND ADMINISTRATION

Preventive care implies a growing organisational function for the doctor, and good administration is necessary to successfully implement preventive care. When designing the practice information system and planning preventive care programmes it is important to ensure that as much as possible of the routine work is delegated to the clerical staff.

SUMMARY

The fact that the general practitioner is responsible for the care of a defined and readily identifiable population gives him the possibility of playing a major part in preventive care. The degree to which he can do this will in large part depend on his willingness to decide on the nature of the care to be provided by the health care team, the attention he gives to developing a suitable information system, and his ability to ensure that optimal use is made of the available resources.

REFERENCES

[1] *Health and prevention in primary care*. Report from General Practice No 18. London: Royal College of General Practitioners, 1981.
[2] Pereira Gray DJ. *Organising preventive medicine. Br Med J* 1982;**284**:709–11.
[3] Stott NCH, Davis RH. The exceptional potential in each primary care consultation. *J R Coll Gen Pract* 1979;**29**:201–5.
[4] Smail SA. Opportunities for prevention: the consultation. *Br Med J* 1982;**284**:1092–3.
[5] Anonymous. Looking after patients with high blood pressure. *J R Coll Gen Pract* 1976;**26**:235–6.
[6] Royal College of General Practitioners. *Computers in primary care.* Occasional paper No 13. London: RCGP, 1980.

Smoking

GODFREY FOWLER

Smoking is the single greatest cause of disease and early death in Britain, and the World Health Organisation has stated that control of tobacco smoking could do more good than any other single action in preventive medicine. At least 50 000 and possibly twice this number of deaths each year in Britain are attributable to it, with an average loss of life of about 10 years. It accounts for about 90% of deaths from lung cancer, 75% of deaths from chronic bronchitis, and 25% of those from coronary heart disease in men under the age of 65 years. But because coronary heart disease is much commoner than lung cancer the actual number of deaths from this cause attributable to smoking is greater than the number of deaths from lung cancer. Moreover, the risk of coronary heart disease attributable to smoking is greater in the younger age group, so that a man under 45 years who smokes 25 or more cigarettes a day may have a 15 times greater risk of dying from a heart attack than if he were a non-smoker.[1]

Advice to stop smoking is the most important help the doctor can offer the patient who has bronchitis, ischaemic heart disease, intermittent claudication, or peptic ulcer. The effects of smoking on health may be summarised as follows:

—Smoking causes many diseases, notably lung cancer, chronic bronchitis and emphysema, coronary heart disease and peripheral arterial disease.

—Furthermore, in pregnant women it has harmful effects on the fetus.

—Children are harmed by parental smoking—directly and by encouragement to smoke themselves.

—Passive inhalation of tobacco smoke by non-smokers is harmful to them.

—The risk of harmful effects from smoking is reduced by stopping smoking, and the benefits occur remarkably quickly in the case of coronary heart disease.

—The switch from plain to filter cigarettes has reduced the risk of lung cancer but not the risk of heart disease (which it may even have increased).

PREVALENCE OF SMOKING

There have been big changes in smoking in Britain over the past 30 years, particularly during the past decade. In the early 1950s almost two thirds of men (and two fifths of women) were regular cigarette smokers, while now just over 40% of men and just under 40% of women smoke. This decline in smoking is largely due to changes in the social class pattern of the habit. In 1960 smoking in men was more or less equally common in all social classes, but by 1972 the proportion of social class V who smoked was almost double that of social class I and now it is almost treble. Translation of this behavioural change among professionals to the population as a whole is the most important challenge facing preventive medicine. Doctors have been particularly successful in stopping smoking, 80% now being non-smokers (and 40% ex-smokers), and this enhances their potential to help others to stop.[2]

There have also been changes in the type of cigarettes smoked. Over 90% of cigarettes now sold are filtered, and there has been a substantial reduction in the tar yield of both plain and filter cigarettes. But while this has reduced the carcinogenic effect of smoking there is no evidence that filters reduce the risk of coronary heart disease and there is even some suggestion that they may be worse in this respect than plain cigarettes. It also appears that smokers adjust their smoking habits to compensate for "weaker" cigarettes—a change to lower tar cigarettes being accompanied by more intense inhalation.

STOPPING SMOKING—THE ROLE OF THE GENERAL PRACTITIONER

Surveys show that most smokers—at least 70%—want to stop smoking. Eighty per cent claim that they would stop if advised to do so by their doctors, but only 10% say that they have ever been advised to do so, despite the fact that most doctors think that this is an important task.[3] Each general practitioner has on his list on average at least 600 patients who smoke, two thirds of whom consult him at least once a year. The scope for offering help is therefore considerable, especially as advice by the general practitioner backed up with a leaflet and follow up has been shown to help patients to stop smoking. In a controlled trial Russell *et al* showed that such advice as part of a routine consultation in general practice resulted in about 5% of smokers giving up—representing about 25 ex-smokers a year for the average general practitioner or over half a million for all 25 000 general practitioners (figure).[4]

The role of the general practitioner in helping patients to stop smoking is therefore to: (*a*) ask about and record patients' smoking habits; (*b*) offer advice when requested; (*c*) seek an opportunity to offer advice in any consultation; (*d*) advise on how to stop; (*e*) supplement advice with appropriate literature; (*f*) follow up patients' attempts to stop; (*g*) set a good example by not smoking—at least in front of patients.

The advice offered should be in the context of the presenting

Smoking

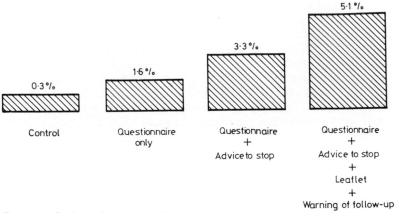

Percentage of patients who gave up smoking.

medical problem when possible and should include: (*a*) information about the health hazards of smoking; (*b*) emphasis on the benefits of stopping smoking; (*c*) a reminder that there is no panacea and that motivation is important; (*d*) a plan to include a target date for stopping; (*e*) advice on ways to prepare for stopping; (*f*) advice on how to cope with difficulties after stopping; (*g*) a warning about the dangers of relapse; (*h*) explanation of the need for follow up.

GUS KIT

The GUS Kit is a literature pack that has been specially designed for general practitioners to help their patients to give up smoking. Produced by Action on Smoking and Health (ASH) in conjunction with the Health Education Council (HEC) and the Scottish Health Education Group (SHEG), it has been circulated to all general practitioners. The kit consists of posters, a guide for general practitioners, notes for receptionists, and a patient booklet. The most important feature is the patient booklet, which is designed to look like and be used like a National Health Service prescription, so that, like the latter, it may be made personal to the particular patient.

NICOTINE CHEWING GUM

Nicotine chewing gum has recently become available on prescription only (but not on the National Health Service), and its usefulness is being evaluated. There are two ways in which it may help: by providing a substitute oral activity and by relieving withdrawal symptoms owing to nicotine dependence. Careful attention needs to be paid to instructions on how to use the gum (a useful leaflet is available from the manufacturers of Nicorette) and its use probably needs to be

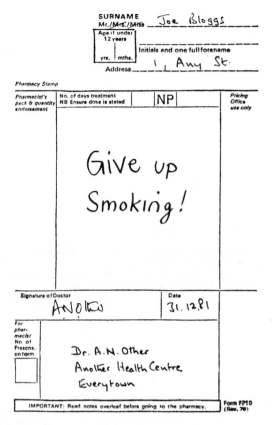

SURNAME
Mr./Mrs./Miss ___Joe   Bloggs_____

Age if under
12 years

Initials and one full forename

yrs. mths.   1, Any St.

Address_____

Pharmacy Stamp

Pharmacist's pack & quantity endorsement	No. of days treatment NB Ensure dose is stated	NP	Pricing Office use only

Give up
Smoking!

Signature of Doctor   Date
ANOther   31.12.81

For pharmacist No. of Prescns. on form

Dr. A.N. Other
Another Health Centre
Everytown

IMPORTANT: Read notes overleaf before going to the pharmacy.

Form FP10
(Rev. 78)

continued for about three months. For most smokers the 2 mg (rather than the 4 mg) strength seems appropriate.

The results of early studies have suggested that it is more effective than other methods of helping people to stop smoking.[5] It may be especially useful for those smokers who have tried other methods without success and who may be presumed to be dependent on nicotine. Use of the gum may enable such smokers to tackle smoking in two stages—first the habit and then the nicotine dependence.

OTHER METHODS

Many other techniques such as hypnosis, acupuncture, aversion therapy, rapid smoking, and group therapy have been tried.[6] Some individuals benefit from such approaches, but there is no scientific evidence that any one of these methods is better than another—or better than firm personal advice from the general practitioner (backed up with a booklet).

Smoking

ACTION REQUIRED

Ask about smoking and record it in notes routinely.

Inform smokers of the risk of continuing and the benefits of stopping.

Offer advice on how to stop and help patients in doing so.

Set a good example.

Prohibit smoking on surgery or health centre premises.

The GUS Kit and bulk supplies of the GUS patient leaflet are available free from the Health Education Council, 78 New Oxford Street, London WC1A 1AH.

REFERENCES

[1] Doll R, Peto R. Mortality in relation to smoking: 20 years' observation of male British doctors. *Br Med J* 1976;ii:1525–36.
[2] Department of Health and Social Security. *Smoking and professional people*. London: HMSO, 1976.
[3] Jamrozik KD, Fowler GH. Anti-smoking education in Oxfordshire general practices. *J R Coll Gen Pract* 1982;**32**:179–83.
[4] Russell MAH, Wilson C, Taylor C, Baker CD. Effect of general practitioners' advice against smoking. *Br Med J* 1979;ii:231–5.
[5] Raw M, Jarvis MJ, Feyerabend C, Russell MAH. Comparison of nicotine chewing gum and psychological treatments for dependent smokers. *Br Med J* 1980:**281**:481–2.
[6] Smoking and how to stop. *Which?* Aug 1980:473–7.

Hypertension

JOHN COOPE

Preventing stroke and heart failure depends on identifying rises in blood pressure in the asymptomatic stage. This requires systematic detection and follow up of patients in general practice. A method for doing this and classifying patients into one of three groups is described.

The case for anticipatory care is nowhere better proved than in the treatment of hypertension. To wait for the patient to present with symptoms today is simply bad medicine. The "rule of halves" indicates that for every patient identified with seriously raised blood pressure there is another in the community who is unidentified. Of those patients who are known to be hypertensive, only half are treated, and of these, only half are adequately treated.

A middle aged man came down to the medical centre to have his ears syringed. My partner noticed a circular disc on the record envelope and asked him whether she might take his blood pressure. His diastolic pressure was 170 mm Hg. Apart from his deafness he felt very well. All practices that do not screen for hypertension will have patients with seriously raised pressures who are not on treatment, and nine out of 10 will visit the medical centre over a period of three years. The need is obvious. How is it to be met?

FIRST SCREEN THE RECORDS

The Achilles heel of much work in practice is the records system. It is a disheartening and difficult place to start. But unless the records have some semblance of order most of the information that is collected for ongoing care will be lost. Many patients, particularly women, will already have a record of blood pressure in their notes as part of a routine examination for issuing the contraceptive pill or for menopausal symptoms. Measuring and recording the pressure, however, is not always followed by taking appropriate action. We found not a few cases in which unacceptable levels of blood pressure had been recorded and not followed up—both in the continuation notes and in hospital letters. Other patients had been established as hypertensive in the past and started on treatment but had failed to continue with it. A 56 year old man with a right partial hemiparesis from birth who had been on treatment for severe hypertension had not attended the surgery for three years. When sent a card he came along readily, and when asked why he had not attended said he felt quite well and thought he had been cured. Had he really not got the message or were his tablets giving him unpleasant side effects which he did not feel like

Hypertension

owning up to? Or was he just a "don't care" type? It was difficult to be sure, but such cases are very common. New patients will be joining the practice list and as their records arrive this is a good time to see whether there is a satisfactory record of blood pressure. We start looking systematically for hypertension at the age of 35, and this means that one new section in the age-sex register comes under surveillance each year and those patients should have their cards examined.

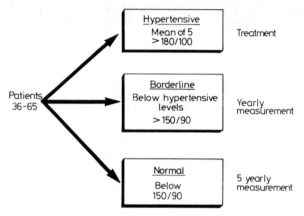

Classification of blood pressure. The three box system.

Recording ongoing information in the same place in the envelope is obviously very useful. We use the reverse side of a problem list card, but there are many variations on this theme. For the past year we have employed a nurse-receptionist whose role is to perform a "Forth Bridge" type maintenance operation on the practice records. She sorts and weeds letters, arranges continuation cards in order, and, if blood pressure checks are required, draws them to my attention. If there is no record whatever of blood pressure (especially in the case of middle aged men) or if there are hypertensive levels recorded, I ask her to send the patient a card asking him to attend the practice nurse for blood pressure examination. Most come. If the situation is less urgent she writes "Take Blood Pressure" on the next line of the continuation card. I find this less likely to be ignored than stickers on the front of the envelope.

Starting from the medical record in this way a continuous screening programme may be planned with the object of recording the blood pressure of every patient on the practice list at least every five years between the ages of 35 and 65.

CLASSIFYING BLOOD PRESSURE

At this point the problem of the variability of blood pressure raises its ugly head. Some patients will be found with what look like treatable levels but which, on repeat takes, seem to return to normal over a few weeks. In others the pressure hovers around a level such as 160/95, where we may not think it justifiable to subject the patient to treatment but do not want to leave the matter for five years without review. These constitute an important borderline group, and we review them yearly. We define the group in terms of at least one pressure over 150 mm Hg systolic or 90 mm Hg diastolic but not high enough to warrant treatment. At first we simply asked them to book an appointment in a year's time but most forgot. We now keep a card index file of these patients and send for them in rotation to attend a clinic run by the practice nurse in the evenings. When the clinic was held during the day large numbers of working patients failed to turn up.

Patients with borderline rises in blood pressure will be additionally at risk if they have other risk factors. Smoking and obesity may be tackled at this stage. A bad family history or diabetes may lower our threshold for treatment. I recently waited too long in a 52 year old patient with diabetes who, after being followed up for some years at the borderline clinic, was found to have a mean blood pressure over five readings of 187/109. He did not attend for six months after these readings so he was sent for with the object of starting him on treatment. When he attended his pressure was 146/90. At the same time he had some new vessel formation in the right eye and was referred to an ophthalmologist. He was reluctant to have blood pressure treatment and asked if he could try weight reduction and come again for review. Six weeks later he had not managed to reduce his weight and his pressure was 186/100. He was also due to have an operation for an inguinal hernia and again asked me to defer a decision on treatment while he made fresh efforts to reduce weight. I agreed, but unfortunately two months later he had a major right hemiplegia. This case shows well the difficulty of making decisions and of sticking to them in the face of pressures from patients who often fear long term treatment.

It is worth asking patients with borderline rises about salt intake and alcohol consumption. Heavy salt users will readily admit to this on questioning and should be told that it pushes up the pressure and to try to get used to food without adding salt at table. Patients who drink more than six pints of beer a day or the equivalent are also increasing their blood pressure and should be counselled, though this habit may be difficult to alter.

Hypertension

The decision to put patients on treatment for hypertension is a serious one for the patient and the doctor. It should not be made in a hurry, and it should be accompanied by a very full explanation. Because of the natural variability of blood pressure, sufficient base line readings should be obtained. I use a minimum of five. These are done by the practice nurse who refers the patient for treatment if the mean systolic pressure exceeds 180 or the diastolic 100 mm Hg. A separate card index file is kept for treated hypertensives. This is examined every three months to make sure that patients are attending. Tagging age-sex register cards or computer recall systems may be used for the same purpose. If no system is used sooner or later patients will stop attending.

CONCLUSION

Classifying patients into three groups or "boxes," as shown in the figure, enables follow up of blood pressures to be organised rationally in a practice. They key to the whole operation is the education and motivation of the nurse. It is she who will be doing most of the blood pressure estimations and maintaining the card index files and ensuring that patients continue to attend. Ultimately it will be with her that they will develop the close rapport that is essential for the prevention of disease in symptomless patients.

Contraception

M J V BULL

It has been suggested that the future health of populations depends more on using preventive measures than on advances in therapeutics; that the best way of introducing prophylactic practices is through health education; and that the latter (in Britain, at any rate) may most effectively be achieved by family physicians.

Twenty per cent of patients in Britain are women in their child bearing years, and it is likely that most will at some time require advice concerning fertility control. The doctor is thus presented with a well motivated group of patients for whom advice concerning contraception may be related to health education and also used to implant attitudes and practices that may benefit both the patient and her family for many years.

THE FIRST CONSULTATION

The first visit that the patient makes to the general practitioner will mainly be concerned with a general discussion of fertility control and the choice of an appropriate method. The table lists some factors that may be considered. A basic philosophy might be:

—hormonal contraception, which has a high degree of reliability, aesthetic acceptability, and reversibility, will be the method of choice before childbearing;

—the intrauterine device, which requires low compliance but is reasonably reliable, may be most appropriate for spacing births;

—sterilisation of one or other partner may be most acceptable when the family is complete, although the woman may still have 15 or 20 fertile years ahead.

Not every patient of course will accept this policy, and an informed decision concerning the most appropriate choice must be made and personal wishes accommodated in each case. It is reasonable, however, to assume that 90% of women presenting for the first time will request a hormonal method (probably the combined oestrogen/progestogen pill), and the stage will be set for a review of current health together with future supervision and screening. The procedure for starting medically supervised contraception will now be described, but, since the all important initial interview is necessarily time consuming, many practices allocate a special session for this purpose. Including a family planning nurse in the primary care team will greatly facilitate examination, instruction, and subsequent supervision of patients at this clinic.

The initial consultation will form the data base for the future care of

Contraception

Factors that influence the selection of the method of contraception

Method	Reliability of method	Compliance required	Aesthetic acceptability	Reversibility	Potential morbidity	Medical initiation	Continuous supervision
Rhythm	Poor	Very high	Good	Good	No	(Yes)	No
Spermicide alone	Poor	Very high	Poor	Good	No	No	No
Condom	Good	Very high	Poor	Good	No	No	No
Diaphragm	Good	Very high	Poor	Good	No	Yes	(Yes)
Intrauterine device	Good	Low	Good	Good	Yes	Yes	Yes
Hormonal method:							
Combined pill	Very good	High	Very good	Good	Yes	Yes	Yes
Progestogen only	Good	Very high	Very good	Good	Yes	Yes	Yes
Vasectomy	Very good	Nil	Very good	Very poor	Yes	Yes	No
Tubal occlusion	Very good	Nil	Very good	Poor	Yes	Yes	No

the patient, and it may be appropriate to use a special record that will be both a primary check list and a flow chart for subsequent observations.

Medical history

The patient's personal history should record major illnesses, accidents, and operations and complications, particularly venous thrombosis and blood transfusion. Inquiries should also be made concerning congenital defects—for example, cardiac or metabolic—recent liver dysfunction, migraine, epilepsy, and sexually transmitted disease. Smoking habits and family history (cerebrovascular accident or myocardial infarction in close relatives) should be recorded, and the implications for the chosen contraceptive method and the patient's health in general may then be discussed. Menstrual and obstetric history is important, and the impact of the chosen method on cycle control and future fertility should be considered.

Physical examination

Height and weight should be measured and the norm for age estimated. Dietary advice may be appropriate. The cardiovascular system should be examined with special emphasis on blood pressure and heart sounds (to detect congenital defect or valvular disease), and the state of leg veins noted. The respiratory system should be examined and appropriate advice given to patients with chronic respiratory disease and to smokers. The breasts should be checked for overt pathology and, for older women, advice regarding self examination may be appropriate. Examination of the genital tract should include the vagina: any congenital defect or evidence of infection? the cervix: any erosion, polyp, or other overt pathology? the uterus: size, position, fibroids, etc; the adnexal organs: any abnormal masses or tenderness?

SPECIAL INVESTIGATIONS

The urine should be examined for sugar and protein. If either is present appropriate investigations should be arranged. Certain blood tests may also be appropriate. Women of Negro or Mediterranean origin should be screened for haemoglobinopathies. Identifying the patient's blood group and rhesus status is also important (if rhesus negative) in the event of subsequent trauma or miscarriage. Rubella immunity status should be ascertained, and seronegative women should be vaccinated once effective contraception has been started. Women with a history of jaundice, pruritus gravidarum, or suspected drug abuse should be screened for HBAg status, and biochemical tests of liver function should also be done since oestrogens should not be

Contraception

used if there is evidence of impairment. A chest x-ray examination should be arranged for recent immigrants and patients with a history of chronic respiratory disease.

Although cervical cytology is an important screening procedure for the future, there is little logical reason for performing this on every teenager starting contraception. A more sensible policy is to start cytological testing when the woman has been sexually active for two to three years. A second smear should then be performed one year later to exclude a false negative on the first occasion. Thereafter, repeat cytology may conveniently be combined with systematic examinations at intervals (see below).

IMPLEMENTATION

The *"pill"*—The mode of action and method of administration must be explained. Possible side effects and problems—for example, breakthrough bleeding, amenorrhoea—should be discussed and questions answered. An appropriate formulation should be prescribed and an appointment arranged for a review.

The intrauterine device—The mode of action and how the device is fitted should be explained and early side effects, such as menorrhagia and discomfort, discussed. A suitable appliance is selected and an appointment for insertion made.

The diaphragm—The method of use is explained and the required size determined. The patient must be instructed in how to place it correctly, how to use the spermicide, and how to care for the appliance.

Sterilisation—Both partners should be interviewed and the method agreed. A full understanding of the procedure is essential, and both tubal occlusion and vasectomy should be regarded as irreversible. Formal consent of both parties will be necessary, together with referral to the appropriate agency.

Other methods—Patients should not only be made aware of how to use the method but of the importance of strict compliance. It would also be appropriate to inform them that in the event of accidental failure or omission postcoital methods of contraception are available provided they are used promptly. For example, Yuzpé's method may be reliably used within 72 hours of risk, or the temporary insertion of an intrauterine contraceptive device may be effective up to twice that time.

CONTINUING SUPERVISION

A planned programme of continuing review for women using any medically initiated method of contraception is advisable since it is over the long term that success must be assured and health education and screening can make its greatest impact. Primarily, satisfaction with the chosen method will be monitored and problems identified and subsequently resolved by modifying the method selected. Appropriate intervals for review (depending on the method used) might be as follows:

The pill—Review after three months, then six monthly. (Check cycle control, symptoms, mood, weight, and blood pressure).

The intrauterine contraceptive device—One, three, six, and 12 months after insertion, then annually. (Check menstrual pattern, pain, bleeding, other symptoms. Pelvic examination for device location.)

The diaphragm—After two weeks, then annually. (Check size, placement technique, and condition of appliance.)

Every five years a major systematic examination should be undertaken, similar to that described above. This may conveniently be linked with the quinquennial birth anniversary (25, 30, 35 years, etc) to remind both doctor and patient when it is next due.

The advantage of an explicit policy for follow up is that the patient becomes accustomed to regular review and examination and will be conditioned to attend when the need for contraception is no longer paramount. Thus as the years pass attendance at the family planning clinic merges into visits to the well woman clinic; the procedures are very similar, apprehension is avoided, and continuing compliance may be achieved. Eventually, screening procedures appropriate to middle and later life can be introduced, degenerative changes anticipated, and continuing health monitored.

FURTHER READING

Anonymous. Screening for cervical cancer in young women. *Lancet* 1978;ii:1029.
Bamford PN. Sterilisation. *Update* 1982;**24**:607–15.
Bluett D. Selection of intrauterine devices. Insertion and removal of IUCDs. *Update* 1981;**22**:165–77, 565–9.
Guillebaud J. *The pill*. Oxford: Oxford University Press, 1980.
Holland WW. Screening and its value. *Update* 1982;**24**:407–17.
Rowlands S, Guillebaud J. Post-coital contraception. *British Journal of Family Planning* 1981;**7**:3–7.

Pregnancy

M J V BULL

The aims of modern maternity care are the early diagnosis of variations from the norm and detection of asymptomatic, potentially
threatening conditions in either mother or fetus. Although systems of
antenatal care are generally well established, it seems likely that they
are not always fully implemented,[1] and opportunities for preventive
care may sometimes be lost. General practitioners, who take some
part in the care of over 90% of pregnant women, are especially well
placed to remedy this.

PRECONCEPTUAL CARE

No woman need conceive before she intends to do so. It has been
shown that premature pregnancy (especially in teenage and unsup-
ported mothers) carries an increased risk of perinatal mortality and
also of subsequent child neglect or abuse. Effective contraceptive
methods should therefore be made available as soon as the need
becomes apparent and the subsequent interval used to prepare the
woman for motherhood. Attendances for fertility control may be used
to educate about smoking, alcohol, drugs, and weight control. When
a woman contemplates becoming pregnant and discontinues contraception nutrition may become important. For example, vitamin B
and folate supplements should be given to any woman with a family or
personal history of a child with spina bifida or anencephaly.[2] Similarly, expatriate Asian women may benefit from vitamin D supplements, since a deficiency has been shown to result in postnatal growth
retardation (and sometimes frank rickets) in the children.

Secondly, preconceptual care may be used for certain relevant
screening procedures. Many schoolgirls born since the 1960s will have
been offered immunisation against rubella in their early teens. Unfortunately, not all took advantage of this opportunity and the
Cendehill-type vaccines that were originally used did not always
achieve satisfactory immunity. Thus even in the 1980s 10 to 15% of
women are seronegative[3] and may thus be at risk of infection during
early pregnancy if they are not identified and immunised at least three
months before contraception is stopped. The blood sample taken for
estimation of rubella haemagglutination inhibition titre may also be
used for ABO and Rh grouping. Rhesus negative women who subsequently abort or terminate a pregnancy should routinely receive anti
D globulin so that the (albeit small) risk of rhesus isoimmunisation is
averted. In women of Mediterranean or African origin the blood
should also be screened for thalassaemia and sickling traits. In Britain

34

about 10% of women of Negro origin are carriers of the HbS gene, and, although they are unlikely to have problems in pregnancy, should they marry a similar carrier the chance of producing a seriously affected homozygous fetus is one in four.

Finally, advantage should be taken during this preconceptual phase to stabilise the management of existing medical conditions, such as diabetes, hypertension, and chronic renal, cardiac, respiratory, or neurological conditions, and to discuss the implications for pregnancy with the patient.

ANTENATAL CARE

Although antenatal care continues to be organised on conventional lines there are certain key points during pregnancy when particularly important procedures should be undertaken.

First consultation

Women should be encouraged to present early in pregnancy to obtain the maximum benefit from the objectives of preventive care. After two menstrual periods are missed it is usually possible to confirm pregnancy by a clinical examination, and specific educational, prophylactic, and screening procedures can begin. If rubella and rhesus status are not already known a blood sample should be taken at the first interview. A patient found to be seronegative for rubella should then be retested three to four weeks later. An appreciable rise in haemagglutination inhibition titre or the presence of IgM antibody suggests recent infection and that termination of the pregnancy must be considered. Part of the first blood sample can also be used for ABO and rhesus blood grouping, and many centres now routinely screen pregnant women serologically for syphilis and hepatitis B. Patients who are seropositive for syphilis should be referred to a specialist in genitourinary medicine, while for hepatitis B carriers special precautions will be required by their attendants during any invasive procedure and at delivery.

Finally, a midstream specimen of urine should be sent for bacteriological examination. About 5% of women will have asymptomatic bacteriuria which, if not treated, may lead to frank pyelonephritis in the mother and possibly an increased risk of retarded intrauterine fetal growth or preterm delivery.

16 weeks

Firstly, is uterine size consistent with gestational age? Estimations based solely on the date of the last menstrual period may be inaccurate in as many as 25% of patients. If a discrepancy exists ultrasonography

Pregnancy

should be requested to enable more accurate dating and to exclude other possibilities, such as missed abortion or multiple pregnancy.

Secondly, at many centres it is now customary to screen all women (with informed consent) for neural tube defects in the fetus. A raised α-fetoprotein concentration in maternal serum detected between 16 and 22 weeks suggests an open neural tube lesion, and a specialist opinion will be needed. Although modern high definition scanners can often show skeletal defects of this type, a high α-fetoprotein concentration in the amniotic fluid is also evidence of an open lesion and an indication for midtrimester abortion.

Amniocentesis should also be offered to any woman with a history of previous chromosomal or neural tube defect or a family history of an enzymatic or sex linked congenital trait.[4] In women aged 37 years and over the probability of the fetus having Down's syndrome becomes greater than the risk to the fetus of amniocentesis, and many patients in this group will request the procedure.

Thirdly, any women with a history of midtrimester abortion (either spontaneous or induced) or previous early preterm delivery should have a careful vaginal examination. Effacement, laceration, or appreciable dilatation of the cervix at this stage may be an indication for cervical cerclage, although the true value of this procedure in the prevention of the preterm delivery has yet to be critically evaluated.

Finally, 16 weeks of gestation is the appropriate time for the patient to receive iron and folate supplements to guard against subsequent development of iron deficiency or macrocytic anaemias of pregnancy. The necessity for these supplements in every case is, however, open to question.[5]

28 weeks

Examination at 28 weeks is of particular importance since it forms a baseline to which deviations from the norm in the third trimester may be related. A blood sample should be checked for anaemia and, in rhesus negative women, for the presence of rhesus antibodies. The gestational age of the fetus should be carefully reassessed on clinical evidence and, if necessary, by ultrasound measurement. Poor maternal weight gain associated with poor uterine growth are important predictors of fetal growth retardation and thenceforth serial ultrasound measurements and maternal urinary oestrogen assays (as indicators of placental function[6]) may be advisable. Women with a history of pre-eclampsia are at risk of both recurrence of this condition and fetal growth retardation, and raised plasma urate concentrations at 28 weeks may predict this. Any history of bleeding in the second trimester is sinister, suggesting placental malposition or abruption. Again, ultrasonography can assist in locating the placenta, and if a low lying placenta can be confidently excluded some degree of abruption should be assumed and specialist opinion sought.

34 to 36 weeks

Maternal blood must again be screened for anaemia and rhesus or other antibodies. Fetal growth should be formally reassessed and investigations started if there is a suspicion of growth retardation. Dynamic tests of fetal wellbeing may now also be appropriate.[7] The simplest is the subjective fetal kick chart, which is completed daily by the mother and should be reviewed at weekly intervals. External cardiotocography may also be advisable; if the fetal heart rate does not react to fetal movement this suggests poor placental function and thus a fetus at risk.

Malpresentation should be obvious by this stage of pregnancy. If a breech or transverse lie is found the advisability of external version must be considered. In nulliparas if version is contraindicated or not feasible a careful clinical and radiological assessment of the pelvis should be made. Any patient whose pelvic architecture is less than optimal may better be delivered by elective lower segment caesarean section. On the other hand, when the presentation is cephalic, cephalopelvic disproportion need rarely be considered before the patient is in labour.[8]

Finally, infective agents in the birth canal may threaten the infant during parturition. In any women with a past history of herpes genitalis, a high vaginal swab should be taken and sent in transport medium for virological examination. If herpes virus is detected delivery may be achieved more safely abdominally than vaginally. Similarly, since perhaps one in eight women is an asymptomatic vaginal carrier of group B streptococcus, and the incidence of streptococcal septicaemia in neonates is 2 per 1000, there may be a case for investigating all patients bacteriologically at 36 weeks and treating the offspring of positive women with prophylactic antibiotics.

One week past term

Perinatal mortality increases with the duration of postmaturity. Evidence regarding accuracy of gestational dating should be reviewed in any woman who is still undelivered one week past term. If no reasonable doubt exists regarding her dates induction of labour should then be considered.

CONCLUSION

The main causes of perinatal mortality and morbidity today are preterm delivery, congenital defect, and intrauterine hypoxia. Although little progress has been made in either predicting or averting

Pregnancy

the preterm delivery, genetic congenital anomalies can now often be detected and the fetus aborted. Other defects—for example the results of rubella infection in early pregnancy—could, with a sufficiently enthusiastic programme for prophylaxis, be entirely eliminated. Intrauterine hypoxia, presenting as fetal growth retardation, is all too often overlooked but the outcome in terms of fetal wastage could be greatly improved if a higher index of suspicion existed and appropriate management was implemented. General practitioners, in fulfilling their role in the care of women in their fertile years, are in a strong position to initiate the appropriate programmes for prevention and so make an effective contribution toward the health of the next generation.

REFERENCES

[1] Hall MH, Chng PK, MacGillivray I. Is routine antenatal care worthwhile? *Lancet* 1980;ii:78–80.
[2] Smithells RW, Sheppard S, Schorah CJ, *et al.* Apparent prevention of neural tube defects by periconceptional vitamin supplementation. *Arch Dis Child* 1981;**56**:911–8.
[3] Clubb RA, Dove GAW, Macinnes LE, Ind SH. Factors influencing rubella immunity in women. *Br Med J* 1981;**282**:275–7.
[4] Valman HB. Amniotic fluid investigations. *Br Med J* 1979;ii:1272–3.
[5] Smail SA. Dietary supplements in pregnancy. *J R Coll Gen Pract* 1981;**31**:707–11.
[6] Shaxted EJ. The use of urinary oestriol estimation. *Journal of Maternal and Child Health* 1981;**6**:325–9.
[7] Godfrey KA. Fetal monitoring in pregnancy and labour. *Practitioner* 1981;**225**:1253–9.
[8] O'Driscoll K, Meagher D. *Active management of labour. Clinics in obstetrics and gynaecology.* Suppl 1. London: W B Saunders, 1980.

Alcohol

PETER ANDERSON

During the past 20 years alcohol consumption in Britain has roughly doubled. In 1980 the British population spent £10 200m—7·5% of consumer outlay—on alcohol, drinking the equivalent of nine pints of beer a week for each individual over the age of 16. Associated with the increase in consumption there has been an increase in the many forms of individual and social damage related to alcohol abuse. The Office of Health Economics estimate that 150 000 people, or 0·4% of the total adult population, are dependent on alcohol; 700 000 (2%) have problems related to alcohol; and 3 000 000 (8%) are heavy drinkers, showing detectable biochemical abnormalities. The number of premature deaths due to alcohol in Britain is probably about 5000 to 10 000 a year.

ROLE OF THE GENERAL PRACTITIONER

General practitioners have special opportunities for helping patients with alcohol problems because they are ideally placed to recognise the problem early and intervene. In terms of prevention we should concentrate on the heavy drinkers rather than the alcohol dependents. Most people who are dependent on alcohol only present for help around their mid forties, after 10 to 20 years of heavy drinking during which time help might have prevented the onset of serious difficulties. A general practitioner with 1800 adult patients will have 120 heavy drinkers, 36 with problems related to alcohol, and six alcohol addicts. Because heavy drinkers have more health problems than most people it is likely that they will consult their general practitioner more often.

EFFECTIVENESS OF TREATMENT

General practitioners are frequently pessimistic about the outcome of efforts to help people who are alcohol dependent and problem drinkers. Much of the available data about treatment, however, relate only to samples of severely dependent individuals. Results might be more encouraging in the earlier stages of the cycle, since heavy drinkers are more likely to be able to cut down their drinking than those who are alcohol dependent. Edwards's well known study showed that 50 alcohol dependent men who were treated intensively with all the facilities of an alcohol unit did no better after one year than a control group given only firm advice. Thus a general practitioner can do just as much to help patients with alcohol problems in a short time with simple resources. Although many people with alcohol

Alcohol

problems help themselves, some whose problems remit without specialist intervention attribute the change in their drinking habits to advice from their general practitioner.

AWARENESS OF ALCOHOL PROBLEMS

One difficulty of dealing with alcohol problems is recognising the problem. To help increase one's awareness of patients with alcohol problems it is useful to have a check list or a register of patients at risk (table 1). The physical complaints of heavy drinkers are often vague: loss of appetite, tummy upsets, morning shakes, backache, memory lapses, and accidents. Symptoms of psychological difficulties include unhappiness, erratic moods, sexual failure, family conflicts, and confusion. Social inadequacy is shown by requests for a sickness certificate, underachievement, problems at work, shortage of money, and trouble with the law. The patient must be asked how much he drinks, when, how often, and whether his drinking has ever caused problems. This needs to be done with sympathy and without embarrassment. When the subject is broached most patients appreciate a frank discussion of the role alcohol plays in their lives.

Records are the general practitioner's paper instruments for detecting patients with a drinking problem, and accurate records are important, especially in a group practice where the patient may consult with a different partner. Any suspicion should be recorded in the notes, and the alcohol problem entered on a chronic morbidity register.

SAFE LEVEL OF DRINKING

It is surprising how many people will adjust their drinking habits when it is pointed out to them the difficulties that drinking is causing.

TABLE 1—*Alcohol problem check list*

Accidents	*Occupations*
Work, home, road	Catering trade
	Publicans
Alcoholic symptoms	Seamen
Smelling of alcohol at consultation	
Morning shakes	*Physical symptoms*
Memory losses	Gastrointestinal upset—pain, vomiting,
Withdrawal fits	diarrhoea
Known alcoholic	Obesity, especially in men
Blood tests	*Psychological symptoms*
Raised mean cell volume, particularly	Anxiety
above 98 fl	Attempted suicide
Raised γ-glutamyltranspeptidase,	Depression
particularly above 50 IU/l	Sexual problems
Family	*Social*
Psychological problems in spouse	Criminal offences
Psychological problems in children	Financial problems
Battering of wife or child	Work problems

This is particularly so of those who have developed a medical problem that is instantly made worse by drinking and so reminds them constantly of the need to change their drinking habits. It is necessary to tell people what is a safe level of drinking. The Royal College of Psychiatrists recommended that the equivalent of four pints of beer was the uppermost acceptable daily intake. But this was designed to stop an individual developing dependence or cirrhosis of the liver, and damage may result from drinking much smaller amounts. A more acceptable level may be the equivalent of two or three pints of beer two or three times a week.

GENERAL PRACTITIONER'S ADVICE

Individuals must be made aware of the health hazards of drinking since heavy drinkers are less aware of the health consequences of drinking than light drinkers (table II). One should also point out that alcohol is an addictive drug and that anyone could, in a given combination of circumstances, become alcohol dependent (table III). Attention needs to be paid to the benefits of reducing drinking rather than to the harm of continuing excessive consumption. One obvious benefit is financial. Others include better judgment and performance, safer driving, and weight loss for obese patients.

Although many people succeed in cutting down their drinking without any help, others need help and the doctor should be willing to help. The advice should be offered not only when requested but also when the opportunity presents in any consultation, especially if it can be related to the presenting medical problem. Literature may reinforce the advice and inform the patient. The Health Education Council has produced two leaflets: *Good Health?* and *Facts about Alcohol*. Further suggested reading is listed.

GOAL OF TREATMENT

The patient has acquired a drinking habit that is damaging his personality, his family, social life, and health. Habits are hard to change and the patient may be ambivalent about changing his drinking pattern. This ambivalence may be met by asking the patient to draw up a balance sheet of the good and bad consequences of his continued drinking, and these may be discussed. Armed with such evidence the patient should set a realistic strategy for changing his lifestyle. It is best to aim for specific short term goals at first so that the patient gets a sense of achievement by attaining, for instance, three weeks' abstinence, or an evening at the pub taking soft drinks. The long term aim for heavy drinkers is to drink less, and a return to controlled social drinking is a realistic aim for a proportion of alcohol dependents.

Alcohol

TABLE II—*Medical conditions related to alcohol*

Accidents

One in three drivers killed on the roads have blood alcohol concentrations over the legal limit. Many accidents at work and in the home are alcohol related.

Brain damage

One in 10 patients in alcohol units has an organic brain syndrome. Shrinkage of the brain can be shown in over half the remaining 90%, many of whom have cognitive impairment on psychological testing.

Cancer

A high alcohol intake increases the incidence of cancer of the mouth, pharynx, and larynx fourfold, oesophagus threefold, and primary hepatocellular carcinoma twofold.

Circulatory system

Moderate consumption of alcohol may decrease the risk of coronary heart disease, but alcohol use increases the risk of raised blood pressure and strokes.

Gastrointestinal

Heartburn, gastritis, and impaired intestinal absorption are common effects of alcohol.

Liver disease

Mortality rates for cirrhosis are 10 times higher in alcohol dependents. Women develop cirrhosis at lower consumption levels than men. Genetic influences probably determine hepatic susceptibility, as not all excessive drinkers develop cirrhosis.

Nutrition

Many moderate drinkers are obese, whereas many alcoholics show evidence of malnutrition.

Pancreatitis

About 25% of all cases of acute pancreatitis are related to alcohol use.

Peripheral neuritis

Develops in 10% of dependent individuals.

Pregnancy

Heavy alcohol intake is associated with the fetal alcohol syndrome. Moderate intake is associated with an increased risk of spontaneous abortion, congenital malformations, and small for dates babies.

Psychological

Alcohol use leads to increased rates of depression and sexual difficulty. Suicide rates in men alcoholics are up to 80 times higher than in non-alcoholics.

CHANGING LIFESTYLE

For many heavy drinkers, drinking has become their predominant interest, and to achieve their desired goal they may have to make major changes in their way of life. The patient will need help to look at impediments to change and alternatives to drinking. Impediments may be a job where drink is readily available, family stress with which the drinker cannot cope without alcohol, or the occurrence of withdrawal symptoms when he tries to stop drinking. The patient should look out for situations and feelings that trigger off drinking and work out new ways of coping with them. To help change their lifestyles patients may be asked to think of activities that they enjoy that do not

TABLE III—*Symptoms of alcohol dependence: typical order of occurrence*

Completely unable to keep to a drink limit
Needing more drink than companions
Difficulty preventing getting drunk
Spending more time drinking
Missing meals drinking
Blackout, memory loss
Giving up interests because drinking interferes
Restless without a drink
Changing to same drinking habits on a work day as on a day off
Organising day to ensure supply
Change to drinking same amount whatever mood
Passing out while drinking in public
Trembling after drinking day before
Times when can't think of anything but getting a drink
Morning retching or vomiting
Sweating excessively at night
Withdrawal fit
Morning drinking
Decreased tolerance
Waking up panicking or frightened
Hallucinations

involve drinking. Alternatives may become clearer if specific attention is paid to past events that triggered drinking—for example, the prematch drink may be avoided by meeting at the football ground.

FAMILY

The family will need help in supporting the problem drinker. The family may feel confused, bitter, and devalued and will welcome the chance of being understood and participating in the process of recovery.

REVIEW

Whatever the agreed goals it is essential to review the patient's progress and to offer continuing help and support and advice on managing difficulties. A diary in which the patient makes a note of any drinks consumed, the time, the quantity, and the occasion is useful for self audit. Supportive laboratory tests (mean cell volume, blood alcohol, and γ-glutamyltranspeptidase concentrations) are useful to monitor progress, and the results and their implications may be discussed with the patient.

RELAPSE

Most patients will drink again whatever the original goal of treatment, but this should not be regarded as a loss of all that has been achieved. It should be viewed as an opportunity for the patient to learn more about himself and the problem. Once the relapse has been openly discussed the patient can recognise strategies for preventing a further recurrence.

Alcohol

Drugs have very little place in the long term management of patients with alcohol problems. Drugs may be needed to help withdrawal symptoms for someone who is physically dependent on alcohol. Chlormethiazole in an initial dose of three capsules four times a day, or diazepam in an initial dose of 5 mg four times a day, and both reducing over one week and then stopping, are suitable alternatives. Alcohol sensitising drugs, such as disulfiram or citrated calcium carbimide, have little use, though some patients find them helpful.

REFERRAL

Most heavy drinkers and patients with alcohol problems can be helped by their general practitioner, but there are some whose care the general practitioner may wish to share. Alcoholics Anonymous provides a very supportive self help group. Referral to an alcoholism treatment unit may be needed as much for support of the general practitioner as for the patient. When a patient is referred it is important to maintain a relationship with the patient and to give a further appointment after the initial referral to discuss what took place.

SUMMARY

The role of the general practitioner in relation to drinking is to:
—be aware of problems related to drink;
—offer advice when requested;
—seek an opportunity to offer advice in any consultation;
—advise on how to cut down or stop drinking;
—supplement advice with appropriate literature;
—follow up attempts to reduce drinking.

The advice offered should include:
—reference to the presenting problem when possible;
—information about the safe level of drinking;
—information about the health and personal hazards of excessive drinking;
—information about the nature and meaning of dependence;
—emphasis on the benefit of reducing drinking;
—a plan for a short term goal;
—ways to cope with the difficulties after reducing drinking;
—warning of the dangers of relapse;
—explanation of the need for follow up.

FURTHER READING FOR PATIENTS AND DOCTORS

Alcohol problems: ABC of alcohol; alcohol and alcoholism. London: *British Medical Journal,* 1982. A straightforward guide to helping patients with alcohol problems, and an excellent series by Richard Smith covering the problems of alcohol in Britain.

Alcohol—reducing the harm. London: Office of Health Economics, 1981. An excellent booklet covering the problems of alcohol in Britain.

Alcohol and alcoholism. London: Royal College of Psychiatrists, 1979. A comprehensive account of alcohol problems.

Alcohol and disease. *British Medical Bulletin* 1982;**28**:1. A detailed account of many of the medical and social problems of alcohol.

Alcoholism. Max Glatt. Teach Yourself Books: Care and Welfare Series, 1982. A very comprehensive review of alcohol problems and their treatment.

Alcoholism. Neil Kessel and Henry Walton. Penguin Books, 1969. An easily read account of alcohol problems and their treatment.

Drinking sensibly. London: HMSO, 1981. A discussion document in the prevention and health series.

Women and alcohol. Camberwell Council on Alcoholism, 1980. A comprehensive coverage of the problems of alcohol as experienced by women.

Cancer

ANN McPHERSON

In 1980, 70 000 men and 61 000 women in England and Wales died from cancer. A large proportion of cancers are thought to be environmentally induced. The factors concerned include diet, general lifestyle, chemicals, and other extrinsic agents. Many cancers are thus thought to be, in principle, preventable. Evidence for this is that the rates of onset of certain cancers are changing rapidly; there are large differences in such rates for the same cancers in different countries; likewise, studies of migrants show that they generally develop cancer rates closer to the population they have joined than to those of the genetically similar population in their country of origin.

Cancer accounts for approximately 20% of the deaths in Britain, and cancers of the lung, gut, and breast account for over half of all such deaths. Moreover, the number of deaths from cancer each year has increased over the past 20 years. This is not surprising, however, since the population is aging and cancer is a disease of old age.

Theoretically, of course, most cancers are preventable, but if one thinks about primary prevention smoking is the only important preventable cause of cancer so far clearly identified in Britain and other Western countries. Thus, whereas Doll and Peto[1] have recently calculated that 30% of all cancer deaths in the United States could be avoided by stopping smoking, they estimate that only 3% of people could be saved by avoiding alcoholic drinks, 2% by avoiding obesity, 1% by regular cervical screening and genital hygiene, less than 1% by avoiding inessential medical use of hormones or radiology, less than 1% by avoiding exceptional exposure to sunlight, and less than 2% by avoiding exposure to carcinogens in the occupational context in food, water, or city air. It is likely that similar figures apply to Britain. They also estimated the proportion of cancer deaths attributable to various factors, such as tobacco 30%; diet 35%; alcohol 3%; sexual behaviour 1%.

So, of the most common cancers, lung is the most readily preventable by decreasing tobacco use. Diet is, however, believed to be important in relation to several cancers—for example, colon, endometrium, and breast, with less evidence for ovarian and prostatic cancer. There is growing evidence that diets high in fibre, β-carotene, and retinol A are helpful in avoiding some of these cancers, but there is not yet sufficient evidence for these to be recommended specifically.

WHAT THE GENERAL PRACTITIONER CAN DO

So what role does a general practitioner have in cancer prevention?

In a practice of 2500 it has been estimated[2] that seven or eight new cases of cancer are likely to be seen each year. This would include one case of lung cancer, one of breast cancer, and one of gut cancer. The other four cases would be drawn from a very wide range of other cancers—for example, one case of carcinoma of the cervix every three or four years, one new case of bladder and kidney cancer every three or four years, and one case of cancer of the pancreas and gall bladder every six years. Identifying high risk patients will enable the general practitioner to be selective, both in the area of primary prevention—that is, through offering suitable advice and information—and also in the area of secondary prevention—that is, through performing such screening techniques as routine cervical smears and breast examinations. A fairly intimate knowledge of one's patients is, therefore, a necessary starting point for prevention. Whether they smoke, what their occupation is, or whether a near relative has had breast cancer will indicate what their cancer risks will be and how they can best be helped to avoid them.

Lung cancer

Avoiding unnecessary x-ray investigative procedures is good practice and is directly applicable as primary prevention, but the most obvious issue is that of smoking. Indeed, it might seem that if a patient smokes it is hardly worth discussing other areas of prevention unless the patient is willing to give up that habit. At the very least, all general practitioners in Britain could give antismoking advice, backed up by a simple pamphlet and a promise to check on the patient's progress. At any rate, it is apparent that the medical consultation is one of the few situations in which advice against the habit can be given to individual smokers by a person in a position of authority, though the wider social attitudes are likely to have a greater influence. Moreover, inquiry through personal knowledge of the patient into the reason for smoking may establish why, for example, certain groups of their women patients continue to smoke while more of their men patients are stopping. Doctors obviously cannot make their patients give up smoking, and the blackmail approach suggested by some general practitioners—that they would not treat patients who smoke—is hardly likely to be productive. Nevertheless, giving them the facts—that 25% of all regular cigarette smokers die before their time because of tobacco—and telling them that stopping smoking before they get cancer does make a difference and reduces the risk of dying from tobacco induced diseases, is at least a beginning. Moreover, because of the effects of interaction people who are both heavy smokers and drinkers should be told that they are putting themselves at an even higher risk, not only of lung cancer but also of cancer of the larynx and oesophagus.

Cancer

Cancer of the cervix

The other area in which there is fairly unambiguous evidence for the efficacy of prevention is that of cervical cancer by screening. Cervical cancer is linked with sexual activity, which theoretically makes primary prevention possible but hardly feasible. The use of barrier methods may afford some protection, but immediate prevention of pregnancy may be more important than long term prevention of cancer of the cervix when counselling patients about the method of contraception. Over 2000 women die from cervical cancer each year in England and Wales, and the prevention of these deaths may also be seen as a challenge to general practice. In some countries where cervical cancer screening is routine the reduction in mortality has been dramatic. In the United States and Finland, for example, death rates have been reduced by half in 10 years. In England, however, there has been only a modest fall in the mortality rate.

Most deaths from cervical cancer occur in women aged over 35 and mostly in women who have never had a cervical smear. The debate about who to screen, how often, and where continues, but if all general practitioners ensured that women patients over 35 were screened every five years (for which general practitioners would be paid) there is little doubt that this death rate would be reduced. Each practice can work out how to do it. One may either use consultations for other problems to take a cervical smear or else approach the problem by, for example, identifying all women over 35 and calling them up at five yearly intervals. In practices where this has been done routinely over 80% of women have been screened; by contrast, in other practices this has been achieved for only 10 to 20% of the female population. Young women at risk are perhaps more easily identified as they are seen at antenatal clinics or family planning clinics. Though they must obviously not be forgotten, it is the older women that offer the immediate challenge. Another useful tool here could be a "medicard" which, among other things, would tell each woman when she last had a smear and when the next one was due.

Breast cancer

If preventive action is clearly worth while for smoking and cervical cancer action as regards breast cancer is more controversial. Breast feeding was at one time thought to prevent cancer of the breast, but it has since been shown that this is not so, although early age of first pregnancy offers some protection against this disease. One is really left with screening in an attempt to pick up cases early and so prevent spread and improve outcome. Even at this level it is difficult to know what to advocate in the way of screening. Breast self examination—or "get to know your own breast"—is one possibility, particularly as

48

there is little evidence that general practitioners or nurses are any better at finding lumps. There have been few attempts, however, to evaluate its use and efficacy properly as regards reducing mortality. When attempts have been made to promote it, breast self examination has proved difficult to instigate.

Since early diagnosis probably does give a better outcome in terms of mortality, this is an area where general practitioners could instruct their women patients, especially those with a higher risk of breast cancer—that is, those over 35, those with a mother or sister who has had the disease, and those with previous benign breast disease. In this context it is important to establish a special relationship with the women so that if they do discover a lump in their breast they are not afraid to present. It is only too common for women to be overcome by fear of bad news, fear of wasting the doctor's time, or fear of the possible treatments. Having said this, however, it would be unrealistic to expect people's attitudes to change overnight.

The usefulness of mammography as a routine screening procedure is also not clear cut, though studies in the United States have shown that regular examination by mammography in women over 50 was beneficial in identifying early lesions, which after treatment resulted in a reduction in mortality. Mammography is not available routinely under the National Health Service, however, and financial constraints may well determine its future availability.

Cancerphobia

Finally, there is cancerphobia. The prevention of unnecessary depression and anxiety about cancer is another area in which general practitioners have something to contribute. Just as we have patients who do not believe smoking has anything to do with cancer, so we also have patients who think they will get cancer from using an ironing board with an asbestos stand, from dyeing their hair, or from using fluoride toothpaste. Likewise, the cyclical changes caused by hormones that occur in the breast each month may cause anxiety because of the lumpiness that may occur before menstruation. Thus, general education about cancer can be useful as prevention for psychiatric morbidity.

SUMMARY

Clearly, the opportunities for effective primary or secondary prevention of cancer in general practice are still limited by the dearth of information about aetiology. Primary care has a potentially important part to play in rectifying this, however. We need to carry out studies with epidemiologists to elucidate some of the unknown factors. General practitioners also represent an effective pressure group to

Cancer

bring about environmental changes—for example, getting smoking banned in certain public places. Finally, since we all have our pleasures or bad habits (according to how you view them), general practitioners might be forgiven for thinking that they have to advocate a sober, temperate life with no tobacco, little alcohol, and little sex! We must obviously avoid moralising and do it in a way that is balanced against the fuller pleasures of life, and take into account the fact that stress (engendered perhaps by being told to give up these habits) may itself make us more vulnerable to cancer.

Thanks to Klim McPherson, Phil Strong, and Leo Kinlen for their help.

REFERENCES
[1] Doll R, Peto R. *The causes of cancer*. Oxford: Oxford University Press, 1981.
[2] Fry J. *Common diseases*. 2nd ed. Lancaster: MTP Press, 1979.

Coronary disease

JULIAN TUDOR HART

Though angina was common in the eighteenth and nineteenth centuries myocardial infarction was not recognised and was probably rare. The modern epidemic seems to have begun in the 1930s, about 15 years after the first world war. By the 1950s it was by far the commonest single cause of premature death. Post mortem examinations on soldiers killed in Korea showed that even in men of average age 22 gross coronary atheroma was already present in 77%.[1] Mortality from coronary disease continued to rise after the second world war throughout the industrialised world; between 1951 and 1971 the coronary death rate for men in Britain almost doubled. Coronary disease now accounts for nearly half of all deaths in men before retirement age. As epidemiologists unravelled its major precursors, it began to seem possible that high risks of early death must be an inevitable consequence of general social advance.

CORONARY DISEASE IS NOT INEVITABLE

The view that coronary disease is not inevitable, which associates high risk with good living and consequently links prevention with a shorn, abstinent, and deprived social condition, is now a main obstacle to any serious strategy for controlling coronary disease. Like any effective myth, it contains elements of truth; but in general the concept is false.

This falsity is proved by two incontestable facts. Firstly, within countries (rather than between them) the poor have higher coronary death rates than the rich, with rates 11% above average in unskilled labourers in 1971, and 12% below average in professionals.[2] Social differences in mortality in the younger age groups are much higher than in late middle age. At ages 35 to 44 unskilled labourers are 55% above the mean for the whole population, and professionals are about 75% below it. These social differences are probably the main cause of the large differences between different parts of Britain, with rates in west Scotland, Northern Ireland, and the South Wales valleys 50% higher than in East Anglia and the home counties (fig 1).[3] [4]

The second reason for rejecting a fatalistic view is that in the United States and Australia rates fell by more than 25% in the 10 years from 1968 to 1977, despite a continued rise in general living standards in both countries. The reasons for this fall are still poorly understood. It long precedes mass use of coronary care units or coronary bypass surgery, and even the widespread use of antihypertensive drugs probably contributed little until the mid 1970s in the USA, but the trend

51

Coronary disease

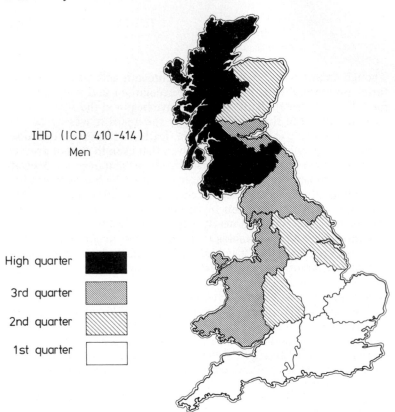

IHD (ICD 410-414)
Men

High quarter
3rd quarter
2nd quarter
1st quarter

FIG 1—Death rates from ischaemic heart disease in men aged 45 to 54, standard regions of England, Wales, and Scotland, divided by quartiles. Reproduced with permission from Fulton *et al. Br Heart J* 1978;**40**;566. ICD=International Classification of Diseases.

does coincide with falls in cigarette consumption and a rise in consumption of polyunsaturated fats.[5] Caution is necessary before concluding that Britain's persistently high rates are attributable to our medical conservatism or the relative poverty of our health service. Rates are stationary also in Sweden, despite excellent high technology services and falling consumption of saturated fats, and rates in American women are falling despite their rising consumption of cigarettes.[6] Both American and Australian rates were a third higher than British rates in 1968, and even now are at about the same level as ours. We still do not know all the major causes of coronary heart disease and sudden heart death, and some of these trends are inexplicable in terms of known risk factors. They do prove, however, that coronary mortality can fall without a nationwide turn to a monastic life.

Coronary disease

The principal known risk factors for coronary disease are cigarette smoking, hypertension, and hyperlipidaemia. There is now no reasonable doubt that these factors are causal and that their control can have some effect on coronary mortality. Other possibly important risk factors are the absence of regular vigorous exercise, having an aggressive and socially ambitious personality, and sustained social or emotional stress. The last two are difficult to define. Nearly all the evidence comes from the USA and may not apply here. Furthermore, there is little convincing evidence that they can be controlled, or that such control reduces the risk of coronary disease. British general practitioners, particularly those in the poorer industrial areas with the worst mortality from coronary disease, have to work very hard at dangerously high speed even to meet the wants of their patients without searching for unmet needs. Any effective strategy for controlling coronary disease in general practice must satisfy two conditions:

(1) Only a few, simple tasks must be required, whose effectiveness must be thoroughly validated by controlled trials. We do not have the time to pursue policies merely because they are rational.

(2) These simple tasks must be made available to everyone at risk in our registered populations, by an active outreach policy.

Only four measures pass this test, all with substantial reservations.

Cigarette smoking

In Doll's study of British doctors[7] men who stopped smoking between 34 and 55 years of age reduced their coronary mortality by half in five years, compared with doctors who continued to smoke. Stopping after 55 made much less difference. About half the benefit of stopping is reached by the end of the first year.[8] The degree of risk is closely related to the number of cigarettes usually smoked,[9] but filter cigarettes are probably not protective.[10] Cigarettes have a synergistic effect on arterial disease with the oral contraceptive pill, increasing the risk of coronary disease (obviously small in young women) twentyfold.[11 12] Stopping smoking after a first infarction is the only measure definitely proved to reduce subsequent mortality from coronary disease, again by about 50% compared with those who continue to smoke.[13–16]

So there is no doubt about the effectiveness of stopping, particularly in young men and women. There is much more doubt about the effectiveness of general practitioners in achieving this end, and more still of their willingness even to attempt it, at least until recently. We are only beginning to learn how to extend the ordinary consultation (for whatever complaint) to include personalised advice on smoking and how to assist people who want to stop, because we are only

53

Coronary disease

beginning to try. The least we can do is to organise our work so that we know the current smoking status of all consulting patients.

Hypertension

Arterial pressure sustained at or above 100 mm Hg (phase 5) through three separate readings should be treated because there is good controlled evidence that this reduces mortality[17] when treatment is begun in middle age. There is no controlled evidence of benefit from treating asymptomatic hypertension in elderly patients. Most of the reduction is by preventing stroke, heart failure, and renal failure. There is persuasive, but so far not conclusive, evidence that antihypertensive drugs, particularly beta-blockers, can also reduce mortality from myocardial infarction.

Controlling borderline hypertension in the diastolic range 90–100 mm Hg, if it was to delete hypertension as a risk factor for coronary disease (perhaps by starting treatment in the 20s or 30s rather than in middle age), would have a far greater potential preventive yield than controlling moderate and severe hypertension of 100 mm Hg+. This is shown clearly in fig. 2.[18] Despite the results of the Hypertension Detection and Follow-up Program in the USA,[19] it is doubtful whether this can or should be done by using antihypertensive drugs, which would require life long medication for 15 to 20% of the adult population. Reducing dietary sodium by a third—from about 150 mmol to less than 100 mmol daily—has now proved effective in controlled clinical trials in hospital patients with borderline hypertension.[20] A similar controlled trial in a free living population is now under way in Glyncorrwg, and it remains to be seen whether it will prove feasible.

Apart from controlling smoking, most of our hopes for future prevention of coronary disease must probably rest on reducing dietary sodium in borderline hypertension. We do not yet know what changes this will imply for general practice, but judging from the poverty of our other token attempts to influence diet in diabetic and obese patients, big changes will be needed, probably requiring large numbers of elementary nutritionists working in the community as members of primary care teams.

Hyperlipidaemias

Severe familial hypercholesterolaemia is rare, causing less than 1% of all hyperlipidaemias. Homozygotes mostly die from coronary occlusion under age 30 unless they are controlled by arduous dieting supported by drugs. With a heterozygote frequency of 1:500, screening of the first degree relatives of every case of coronary occlusion under 50 would detect children at a treatable stage.[21]

54

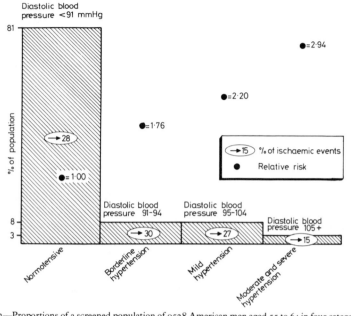

FIG 2—Proportions of a screened population of 9538 American men aged 55 to 64 in four categories by mean diastolic pressure, mean of three readings, from the National Health Examination Survey, 1960–62: and the relative risks of myocardial or brain infarction during one year for the same categories, from the Framingham "blue books." Source: Epstein.[18]

Raised total or low density lipoprotein (LDL) cholesterol increases the risk of myocardial infarction synergistically with the other major risk factors—smoking and hypertension. The association is high in young men and women and declines with age. High density lipoprotein (HDL) cholesterol, on the other hand, protects against coronary disease; it probably reflects cholesterol mobilisation, while LDL cholesterol reflects deposits as athermatous plaque. The protective effect of HDL cholesterol persists in elderly people,[22] but this fraction is influenced more by smoking and exercise than by diet. Consequently, advice about diet needs to be concentrated on people under 50.

There is little evidence that specific cholesterol lowering diets are more effective than diets that aim simply at reducing body weight to within 10% of its ideal level. This can be easily calculated by the formula for body mass index—metric weight divided by the square of metric height. Body mass index should lie between 20 and 25 for adult men and 19 and 24 for women. Triglyceride concentrations, which are also a positive risk factor for coronary disease, are so closely linked to fatness that there is little point in measuring them.

Coronary disease

The safe and effective way to reduce LDL cholesterol is to follow a prudent diet, with calories restricted to attain ideal weight, all fats reduced from a current 40% to about 30% of total calorie intake, and more high residue foods. It is probably sensible to replace as much as possible of saturated fats with polyunsaturated fats. The disadvantages of clofibrate in promoting gall stone formation probably outweighs any advantages. Shifts in dietary habits leading to a reduction of LDL cholesterol are probably occurring now because of changes in public opinion about the wholesomeness of foods. In 1980 the consumption of sugar in Britain went down by 8%, eggs by 10%, milk by 10%, white bread by 20%, and butter by 22%; whereas consumption of potatoes rose by 23%, margarine by 27%, and brown bread by 41%.[23] All the indications are that people are able and willing to change, but in addition to needing better, informed help from their own doctors, food manufacturers will have to make labels more informative and less promotive. Perhaps as a profession we need to press for the legislation to secure such a change.

Exercise

Retrospective studies tend to show lower coronary risks for those who take vigorous daily exercise, though the differences are less than those attributable to smoking, hypertension, or hyperlipidaemia.[24-26] Such people, however, obviously differ from those who make other uses of their leisure time. Controlled prospective studies of exercise programmes after myocardial infarction in people under 57 showed no improvement in survival after four years, though fitness as measured by a bicycle ergometer was appreciably improved, and effort tolerance in those with angina had increased 100%.[27]

Regular exercise, however, could have an important indirect effect on other, more potent risk factors by providing an essential part of a more general changed lifestyle emphasising active creativity rather than passive consumption. Much more needs to be done to link primary care with local sports facilities (as in the siting of health centres at Milton Keynes new town) to assist those over 30 to acquire or maintain non-competitive sporting activity.

A PLAN FOR GENERAL PRACTICE

Looking at the whole field of atheromatous arterial disease, stroke as well as coronary occlusion, the Royal College of General Practitioners working party on prevention[28] recommended immediate action on three points for the whole adult population up to age 65: (*i*) control of hypertension when the diastolic pressure is 105+ (which we would now reduce to 100 mm Hg in the light of the Australian trial); (*ii*) personalised advice on smoking; and (*iii*) measurement of weight and

56

height in all who look fat, calculation of ideal weight, and advice and support for those who want to try to attain it. Three further points for immediate action were suggested for subgroups: known diabetic patients should be reviewed for other coronary risk factors, particularly smoking and hypertension, and diet should be reviewed to reduce the total amount of fat; women on oral contraceptive pills should have their arterial pressure monitored regularly and be advised on smoking; and the need for thiazide diuretics should be reviewed regularly to avoid unnecessary use of these eventually diabetogenic drugs.[29 30]

We have to start from where we are. Half our hypertensive patients are unknown, and half of those who are known are not controlled. Our diabetic patients seem to be equally divided between those who receive impersonal—and therefore inefficient—hospital care, those who see their general practitioners but receive little effective monitoring, and those who pick up repeat prescriptions but receive no regular medical supervision.[31] *Step one* for every practice that is seriously interested in preventing coronary disease must surely be to improve the quality of care and follow up of these two very high risk groups. Few of them rightly belong in hospital outpatient departments, for their clinical needs are simple—regular monitoring of arterial pressure and search for side effects of drugs for hypertensive patients and regular monitoring of optic fundi, glycosylated haemoglobin, and weight for diabetic patients, and sustained pressure to give up smoking for both. *Step two* is to ascertain all hypertensive patients by a regular system of case finding, updated every five years, and to search actively for maturity onset diabetes by screening fat people over 50 for glycosuria, again using case finding. This is likely to double workload in both these categories. *Step three* is to ascertain the smoking status of the whole population aged 12 to 64, and to offer sustained, personalised advice and support in subsequent consultations.

RESOURCES AND ORGANISATION

Preventing coronary disease requires two big changes in practice organisation. Firstly, means must be found to expand the consultation to include an active search for needs as well as the more passive satisfaction of wants. Now, at least in the overworked areas where coronary disease is most prevalent, we have an average face to face consulting time of five minutes.[32] We can do this in three ways: by delegating clinical measurements to employed staff, by taking on more partners whole time or part time, and (doubtfully) by reducing time spent on less useful tasks.

Secondly, we have to make regular monitoring of the whole adult population, or of special groups in it, a normal and necessary part of practice. This requires a record system suitable for such use, with colour tagging, structured display of data, and means of readily identifying tasks not yet done. I do not believe that this can be done within the limits of the Lloyd-George record, and the need to change to A4 has to be faced. It also requires staff time, as well as the support and interest of at least one partner in the group. There can be no greater illusion than that computers will bypass the need for good structured records and substantial staff and medical time devoted to their use. To get beyond our present passive response to breakdown and organise active search for need requires a transformation in the way we work that must precede delegation to machines. Until we have mastered the task it will not be defined or understood, and therefore cannot be computerised. The data inputs will be local, personal, and specific, and can come only from our own work; we cannot buy it off the shelf as computer software.

Our immediate need is more staff, and this should not be a difficulty. Though general practitioners are each entitled to employ two whole time equivalent supporting clerical or nursing staff with 70% reimbursement of wages (and the remaining 30% set against tax), only 15% of all general practitioners currently employ their full entitlement. The average number of staff employed by general practitioners in England and Wales is about 1·2. We seem to be up against our own ancient traditions of counting pennies to let pounds look after themselves—all tactics, no strategy. Except in overdoctored areas, most of us could also get additional medical staff. Preventive work is predictable, crisis free, and could be planned to meet the needs of the growing number of women graduates who need less open ended commitment to practice.

CONCLUSION

The present state of general practice is too variable to permit a cookery book solution for coronary prevention. General practitioners are the most highly educated health workers in their communities. Each of us must adapt, as best we can, the general conclusions of medical science to the specific problems and resources of our local community. Few of us can as yet do all the simple things that need to be done; but even fewer are truly unable to make a start on some of them—not for some, but for all of the people.

REFERENCES
[1] Enos WF, Holmes RH, Beyer J. Coronary disease among United States soldiers killed in Korea. *JAMA* 1953;**152**:1090.
[2] Office of Population Censuses and Surveys. *Occupational mortality 1970–72*. Dicennial supplement No 1. London: HMSO, 1978.

Coronary disease

[3] Fulton M, Adams W, Lutz W, Oliver MF. Regional variations in mortality from ischaemic heart and cerebrovascular disease in Britain. *Br Heart J* 1978;**40**:563–8.

[4] Hart JT. The distribution of mortality from coronary heart disease in South Wales. *J R Coll Gen Pract* 1970;**19**:258–68.

[5] Dwyer T, Hetzel BS. A comparison of trends of coronary heart disease mortality in Australia, USA and England and Wales with reference to three major risk factors. *Int J Epidemiol* 1980;**9**:65.

[6] Marmot MG, Booth M, Beral V. Changes in heart disease mortality in England and Wales and other countries. *Health Trends* 1981;**13**:33.

[7] Doll R, Peto R. Mortality in relation to smoking: 20 years' observations on male British doctors. *Br Med J* 1976;ii:1525–36.

[8] Hammond EC, Garfinkle L. Coronary heart disease, stroke, and aortic aneurysm: factors in etiology. *Arch Environ Health* 1969;**19**:167.

[9] Bain C, Hennekens CH, Rosner B, Speizer FE, Jesse MJ. Cigarette consumption and deaths from coronary heart-disease. *Lancet* 1978;i:1087–8.

[10] Wald NJ. Mortality from lung cancer and coronary heart-disease in relation to changes in smoking habits. *Lancet* 1976;i:136–8.

[11] Mann JI, Vessey MP, Thorogood M, Doll R. Myocardial infarction in young women with special reference to oral contraceptive practice. *Br Med J* 1975;ii:241–5.

[12] Mann JI, Doll R, Thorogood M, Vessey MP, Waters WE. Risk factors for myocardial infarction in young women. *Br J Prevent Social Med* 1976;**30**:94–100.

[13] Hammond EC. Smoking in relation to disease other than cancer. In: Richardson, ed. *Second world conference on smoking and health*. Bath: Pitman Press, 1972:24.

[14] Gordon T, Kannel WB, McGee D, et al. Deaths and coronary attacks in men after giving up cigarette smoking. *Lancet* 1974;ii:1345–8.

[15] Wilhelmsson C, Vedin JA, Elmfeldt D, Tibblin G, Wilhelmsen L. Smoking and myocardial infarction. *Lancet* 1975;i:415–20.

[16] Mulcahy R, Hickey N, Graham I, McKenzie G. Factors influencing long-term prognosis in male patients surviving a first coronary attack. *Br Heart J* 1975;**37**:158–65.

[17] Report by the Management Committee. The Australian therapeutic trial in mild hypertension. *Lancet* 1980;i:1261–7.

[18] Epstein FH. An epidemiological view of mild hypertension. In: Gross F, Strasser T, eds. *Mild hypertension: natural history and management*. London: Pitman Medical, 1979:3–13.

[19] Hypertension Detection and Follow-up Program Cooperative Group. Five-year findings of the HDFP. I Reduction in mortality of persons with high blood pressure, including mild hypertension. *JAMA* 1979;**242**:2562–71.

[20] McGregor GA, Markandu ND, Best FE, et al. Double-blind randomised crossover trial of moderate sodium restriction in essential hypertension. *Lancet* 1982; i: 351–5.

[21] Slack J. *Early metabolic prediction in adults*. Amsterdam: Excerpta Medica, 1978:111.

[22] Gordon T, Vastelli MP, Hjortland MC, et al. High density lipoprotein as a protective factor against coronary heart disease. *Am J Med* 1977;**62**:707.

[23] Richardson DP. Changing public ideas about the wholesomeness of food. *Nutrition Bulletin* 1982;**7**:31.

[24] Morris JN, Chave SPW, Adam C, Sirey C, Epstein L, Sheehan DJ. Vigorous exercise in leisure-time and the incidence of coronary heart disease. *Lancet* 1973;i:333–9.

[25] Paffenbarger RS, Hale WE. Work activity and coronary heart mortality. *N Engl J Med* 1975;**292**:545–50.

[26] Kannel WB, Sorlie P. Some health benefits of physical activity: the Framingham study. *Arch Intern Med* 1979;**139**:857.

[27] Wilhelmsen L, Sanne H, Elmfeldt D, et al. A controlled trial of physical training after myocardial infarction. *Prev Med* 1975;**4**:491.

[28] *Prevention of arterial disease in general practice*. Report from General Practice No 19. London: Royal College of General Practitioners, 1981.

[29] Lewis PJ, Kohner EM, Petrie A, Dollery CT. Deterioration of glucose tolerance in hypertensive patients on prolonged diuretic treatment. *Lancet* 1976;i:564–6.

Coronary disease

[30] Amery A, Berthaux P, Bulpit C, *et al*. Glucose tolerance during diuretic therapy: results of trial by the European Working Party on Hypertension in the Elderly. *Lancet* 1978;i:681–3.

[31] Doney BJ. An audit of the care of diabetes in a group practice. *J R Coll Gen Pract* 1976;**26**:734–42.

[32] Buchan IC, Richardson IM. *Time studies in general practice*. Scottish Health Service Studies No 27. Edinburgh: Scottish Home and Health Department, 1973.

Dietary advice

GODFREY FOWLER

Leave gourmandizing; know, the grave doth gape for thee thrice wider than for other men. Shakespeare: *Henry IV*, part II, act V, scene 5.

Historically, malnutrition implied deficiencies in the diet that lead to the traditional deficiency diseases, and this is still the major nutritional problem worldwide. In contrast, however, in this century in some populations diseases of overnutrition have emerged.

"Western diet"—that typical of industrial societies—is thought to contribute to a wide range of "diseases of affluence." These include ischaemic heart disease, diabetes, gall stones, diverticular disease of the colon, irritable bowel syndrome, constipation, appendicitis, large bowel cancer, haemorrhoids, varicose veins, dental caries, and, of course, obesity.

The "Western diet" is characterised by a preponderance of fatty foods, of foods with a high sugar and low fibre content, and an excess of alcohol. Moreover, 75% of food eaten in the United Kingdom is "processed" at least once, which alters the composition and makes identification of ingredients difficult. Such diets commonly include high proportions of sweets, cakes, biscuits, butter, margarine, cream, cooking fats, and fried foods. What bread is eaten is mostly made from white flour. Total energy intake is generally excessive and there is usually also a lot of salt.

During this century the proportion of protein in the diet has remained roughly the same, the proportion of fat has increased (see figure), and that of carbohydrate has fallen—because, although there has been an increase in dietary sugar, less bread and fewer potatoes are eaten. In the past 20 years the proportion of alcohol in the diet has doubled, and this now represents about 5% of the daily energy intake. Originally the prerogative of the richer sections of society, with improved living standards such diets have now become universal in the United Kingdom.

RELATION BETWEEN DIET AND DISEASE

There is accumulating evidence, mostly from epidemiological sources, of the association between dietary excesses and disease.

Coronary heart disease is the major killer in industrial societies. In an early study of the relation between diet and deaths from ischaemic heart disease in seven countries, Keys[1] showed that there were strong positive correlations with the amount of saturated fat and dietary

Dietary advice

sugar eaten and that blood cholesterol concentrations were strongly related to the proportion of calorie intake contributed by saturated fat. Other studies showed that migrating populations, such as Japanese moving to California, in adopting a higher fat diet also acquired a higher incidence of ischaemic heart disease. More recently, the results of intervention studies such as the Oslo Heart Study,[2] a controlled trial in which dietary and smoking advice were studied, have shown a reduction in coronary heart deaths in men who reduced their fat intake. There is also evidence of a positive correlation between coronary heart disease and alcohol intake.

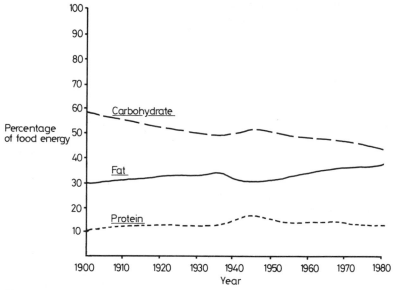

Changes in this century in the proportion of dietary carbohydrate, fat, and protein as a percentage of food energy. Source: *Practising prevention: eating for health.*

Hypertension is associated with obesity, and losing weight leads to a fall in blood pressure. There is also a correlation between salt intake and high blood pressure, evidence that a high intake of salt may cause hypertension in susceptible individuals, and further evidence that reducing salt intake can reverse the process.

Diabetes—the incidence correlates strongly with an excessive intake of energy and fibre may be protective. High fibre diets also improve control of diabetes.

Diverticular disease is associated with a deficiency in dietary fibre and an intake of dietary fibre of 30 g or more a day has been associated with a lower prevalence of diverticular disease. Although no intervention studies have been done to show the protective effect of dietary fibre, the evidence is strong and it has been effective in managing the condition.

Constipation is a common complaint in Western society but rare in countries with high fibre diets and in vegetarians. Increasing dietary fibre increases stool bulk, reduces bowel transit times, and relieves constipation. It also benefits patients with the *irritable bowel syndrome*.

Dental caries is a major problem in the United Kingdom. In a recent survey 80% of 5 year olds required treatment for dental caries and in 10% more than half of their teeth were seriously decayed. On the other hand, caries is rare in countries where food is unrefined.

Gall stones are associated with obesity and there is also evidence that together with *appendicitis* gall stones occur more often in those on a diet that is deficient in fibre.

Obesity is known to have major consequences for health. Much of the evidence comes from life insurance statistics, and there is a clear association between being overweight and premature death from several conditions—from diabetes to accidents. Although obesity arises only when energy intake is greater than expenditure, the problem is not as simple as this. Weight reduction improves life expectancy, lowering blood pressure, among other things.

Cancer is in many instances attributable to aspects of diet. In a recent report Doll and Peto[3] estimated that about one third of all deaths from cancer are attributable to diet—about the same proportion as those caused by smoking. Epidemiological evidence indicates that diet may be important in determining the occurrence of cancer of the stomach, large bowel, uterine body, gall bladder, and liver. It may also contribute to cancer of the breast and pancreas. The mechanisms are unclear, but there is some evidence that dietary fat may be implicated and that β-carotene, the vitamin A precursor, may be protective.

GIVING ADVICE

In the light of these facts, what should the general practitioner do? Firstly, the important role of the general practitioner and other members of the primary health care team, especially the health visitor, in giving such advice must be acknowledged. The Latin derivation of "doctor" is "teacher," and although doctors seem reluctant to see themselves as health educators a recent survey showed that "of all the many and varied sources of health information available to the adult population, it is the general practitioner who is most trusted and whose advice has most impact."

Secondly, advice must be concerned with the broad composition of

Dietary advice

the total diet and must at the same time be specific. Advice should also be reinforced and supplemented with simple literature.

The most important objective is to maintain weight within 10% of the "ideal" or "optimal." This weight (obtained from life insurance data) is that associated with the lowest level of mortality. A useful table is that in *Which? Way to Slim,* which is derived from Metropolitan Life Insurance Tables. Alternatively, body mass index may be calculated. This is the ratio of weight (kg)/square of height (metres) and should be 20–25 for men and 19–24 for women.

Energy requirements vary greatly, but for many this means lowering energy intake by reducing the consumption of sugar and fat. Regular weighing is a necessary corollary.

Advice on individual dietary constituents should include the following:

—*Sugar*: the average individual annual intake of sucrose is almost 100 lb! About half of it is added to beverages, cereals, etc. The amount should be halved.

—*Fat*: many international and national professional and governmental committees have shown a strong consensus that lowering total fat in the diet to about 30% of total energy intake can reduce the risk of coronary heart disease. The debate continues about the relative importance of saturated and polyunsaturated fats, but there is general agreement that dietary saturated fats should be reduced. A reduction in plasma cholesterol concentrations follows such changes.

—*Fibre*: dietary fibre, particularly cereal fibre, is of special interest. To its virtue as a laxative other benefits are now being added, and an intake of 30 g a day from foodstuffs derived from whole grains is recommended. Wholemeal bread and bran rich breakfast cereals are obvious examples, and the increased consumption of both of these is encouraging.

—*Protein*: protein intake in the United Kingdom has remained remarkably stable this century, despite other major dietary changes. There is no evidence to suggest that changes are necessary, though eating less meat as a source of protein and more cereal and vegetable sources of protein incidentally reduce intake of saturated fat.

—*Salt*: the present average salt intake of 12 g a day is excessive and could be halved without detriment and with possible benefit in preventing hypertension.

—*Alcohol*: during the past 20 years alcohol consumption in the United Kingdon has doubled. To preserve health, alcohol intake should not exceed 4% of total calories, which means about 20 g or two "units" a day—the equivalent of two pints of beer or two glasses of wine or measures of spirit.

Dieting is not complicated, and an obsession with calories is unnecessary. The basic rules include: (*i*) a prudent diet with reduced sugar and fat and increased fibre content and less salt and alcohol; (*ii*) regular weighing; (*iii*) avoiding eating between meals—"nibbling" should be of fresh fruit or nuts; (*iv*) awareness of the relation between individual energy intake, expenditure, and storage (fat); (*v*) motivation.

SUMMARY

(1) There should be a simple, standard approach to diet.

(2) The main task is to avoid obesity. Energy intake should be adjusted to maintain optimal body weight (as defined by life insurance statistics or calculations of body mass index).

(3) Average sugar intake should be halved. This means cutting down on sweets, chocolates, puddings, soft drinks, and sweetened beverages.

(4) Fat intake should be reduced to about 30% (from an average now of about 40%) of energy intake and the reduction should be of "saturated" fats. This means cutting down visible fats—for example, butter, margarine, cream, fat on meat, and fried foods.

(5) Intake of fibre should be increased to about 30 g a day (from an average now of about 20 g), and this should be from whole grain cereals.

(6) Salt intake should be halved. Adding salt should be discouraged.

(7) Alcohol intake should be reduced to not more than two "units" (pints of beer/glasses of wine or spirits) a day.

REFERENCES
[1] Keys A. *Seven countries—a multivariate analysis of death and coronary heart disease.* Cambridge, Massachusetts: Harvard University Press, 1980:1–381.
[2] Hjermann I, Hölme I, Velve Byre K, Leren P. Effect of diet and smoking intervention on the incidence of coronary heart disease. *Lancet* 1981;ii:1303–10.
[3] Doll R, Peto R. *The causes of cancer.* Oxford: Oxford University Press, 1981.

FURTHER READING
Department of Health and Social Security. *Prevention and health: everybody's business.* London: HMSO, 1976.
Department of Health and Social Security. *Prevention and health: eating for health.* London: HMSO, 1978.
Department of Health and Social Security. *Prevention and health: drinking sensibly.* London: HMSO, 1981.
Which? Way to slim. London: Consumers' Association, 1978.
Anderson P. Practising prevention: alcohol. *Br Med J* 1982;**284**:1758–60.
Prevention of coronary heart disease: report of expert committee. WHO Technical Report Series 678. Geneva: World Health Organisation, 1982.

FREE LITERATURE
Simple literature on diets: *Fat—who needs it?* and *Fibre in your food* are available from the Health Education Council, 78 New Oxford Street, London WC1A 1AH, and from local health education units.

In old age

J A MUIR GRAY

What are we trying to achieve? This is best answered by the pithy motto of the World Health Assembly's meeting in Vienna in 1982: "Add life to years," and there is evidence that this is what modern medicine manages to achieve. The fear that large numbers of people are being kept alive to a very advanced age by overenthusiastic medical intervention is not supported by demographic data, which show that life expectancy is being increased but not life span. Furthermore, there is some evidence that people are, on average, staying fitter longer and having a shorter period of terminal dependency as a result of the medical, social, and economic changes that have taken place this century. Sir Richard Doll has said that one of his aims in life is to "die young as late as possible," and this is another excellent way of expressing the aims of a prevention programme; the principal aim is to prevent morbidity, not to postpone mortality.

Attention must be focused on the old person's ability to function: a "normal haemoglobin" is of little comfort to someone who is still too breathless to walk to the local pub. The aim of the measures described here is to prevent handicap, and the common handicaps in old age provide a useful list of specific objectives (table I).

TABLE I—*Common handicaps*

Immobility; inability to reach the shops, church, or pub
Inability to dress or undress
Inability to wash all over
Inability to reach the toilet in time
Inability to get enough to eat or drink
Inability to do light housework or gardening
Anything else that the old person regards as a handicap

HOW DO WE ACHIEVE THESE OBJECTIVES?

Although the aging process is not preventable, much can be done to prevent the problems of old age because most of the problems of older people are not caused by the aging process but by one, or more than one, of three other processes—disease, loss of fitness, and the social changes that accompany growing old.

Prevention of disease

The primary prevention of many of the diseases that cause disability in old age is possible, but for most diseases it is necessary to start the preventive programme in childhood or early adult life. This should not be taken as the basis for a nihilistic attitude to disease

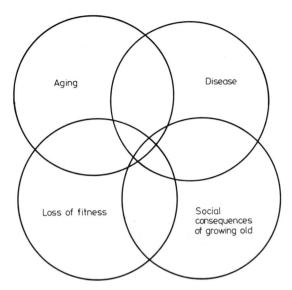

prevention, however, because the diseases listed in table II are preventable by actions initiated after the age of 6o.

The commonest single preventable disease in old age is probably iatrogenic disease, and one of the main contributions that the general practitioner can make to health in old age is to prevent iatrogenic disease by careful prescribing and surveillance of people on repeat prescriptions. Much attention has been given to "poor compliance" recently, but remember that "poor compliance" is often the patient's method of preventing iatrogenic disease.

In addition to measures directed at specific diseases there is also evidence that several measures have beneficial effects on health in old age (table III). Furthermore, body maintenance is of even more importance in old age, for minor disorders of feet, skin, or ears can cause as much suffering as the major illnesses that feature on mortality

TABLE II—*Scope for disease prevention in old age*[1]

Iatrogenic disease
Depression
Anxiety
Alcoholism
Hypothermia
Influenza
Tetanus
Constipation
Some types of fall
Some types of incontinence
Malnutrition

and morbidity statistics. Body maintenance has to be carried out by the individual, but professionals have to teach what should be done and be available when the self help is not working (table IV).

TABLE III—*Scope for health promotion in old age*

(1) Stopping cigarette smoking—has no effect on mortality but has an effect on morbidity
(2) Weight control—avoiding obesity, and weight loss for those who are obese
(3) A prudent diet low in calories, high in fibre
(4) Mental activity and involvement with other people
(5) Keeping fit

TABLE IV—*Scope for body maintenance in old age*

Maintenance programme	The professional's contribution
Foot care	Qualified chiropodist, essential for people with circulatory problems or diabetes
Tooth and denture care	Annual visit to the dentist
Skin care	Treatment of eczema or ulcers; skilled nursing is needed if there are pressure sores
Visual care	Biennial visits to the optician, sooner if vision deteriorates
Hearing care	Auroscopic examination if the elderly patient notices hearing loss

Prevention of unfitness

The older the age group chosen the greater the scope for improving performance by improving fitness because the greater is the size of the fitness gap (fig 1). All four physical aspects of fitness can be improved at any age—strength, stamina, suppleness, and skill. In addition, there are considerable psychological benefits. The steps that may be taken to improve fitness are:

(1) Ensure that there are no diseases present in which exercise would be harmful. There are very few contraindications provided that the person increases his exercise slowly and gently.

(2) Reassure the old person and relatives that exercise will not do harm; the motto is "use it or lose it."

(3) Encourage mobile elderly people to continue with sport and exercise or to take up exercise if inactive. Exercises that promote suppleness are particularly important—swimming, yoga, keep fit, music and movement, and aerobics.

(4) Try to help housebound people reach sports or leisure centres. Give advice on suppleness exercises that can be done at home.

(5) Give advice to relatives and home helps on the health benefits of housework and gardening, especially for the person who finds them a bit of a struggle.

(6) Take an active rehabilitative approach to every immobilising illness. Remember that fitness is lost more easily and regained more

slowly the older you are and the effects of a few days' inactivity may take a few weeks of work to overcome.

The fitness gap is usually bigger—and the scope for improvement therefore greater—when a disabling disease is present because of the immobilising effect of most disabling diseases.

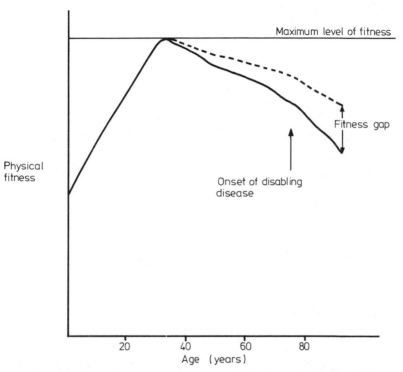

FIG I—Rate of change of physical fitness with age. Broken line = rate of decline due to aging alone if fitness is not lost. Continuous line = actual rate of decline.

Prevention of social problems

Three types of social problems must be taken into account when thinking of prevention in old age. Firstly, elderly people may have very pessimistic and negative beliefs and attitudes.[2] Many believe that all their problems are due to "old age" and ipso facto cannot be prevented or treated. Some are too depressed by their deterioration to try to affect it, and some are too tired by the effort of struggling to summon up the strength to participate in preventive measures. Such people need a very positive approach.

In old age

TABLE V—*Common practical problems*

Poverty
Heating problems
Housing problems
Isolation

Secondly, the beliefs and attitudes of other people have to be taken into account. Many young people are also very pessimistic and nega-

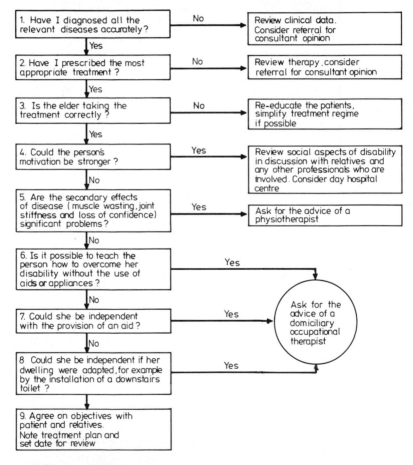

FIG 2—Handicap algorithm: checklist for use when relatives request a service for an old person who has developed a handicap. Always exclude the possibility of a treatable disability before arranging for a service to be given.

tive about the scope for prevention in old age and many are over-protective—some because they are guilty and thus dislike to see an elderly person struggle or be placed at risk. The problems of relatives are more commonly underestimated by professionals than any other single social problem.

Thirdly, the practical problems faced by some elderly people are immense and must always be borne in mind (table V). Obviously doctors cannot solve these problems on their own but they can take three steps.

(1) Know about the range of benefits available.

(2) Be prepared to make the initial contact by phone or letter.

(3) Be prepared to discuss her attitudes with the old person who is unwilling to apply or ask for help.

HOW SHOULD OLD PEOPLE BE REACHED?

Full scale screening is not an efficient approach for reaching old people, and it is more efficient to make full use of the potential offered by any consultation made by the old person or her relatives—the case finding approach, using the exceptional potential of each primary care consultation[3] because most elderly patients will contact the practice at some time during the year. What is needed to make such an approach effective is:

(1) A record and information system that will indicate which patients over the age of 75 have not contacted the practice during the preceding year.

(2) Sufficient data on each patient to indicate which of those who have not made contact need a home visit. These data may be held by the health visitor or in the patient's notes. Rather than having a separate "at risk" register it is better to consider everyone at some degree of risk and have enough data in the notes to allow the identification of those who are at sufficiently high risk to warrant a home visit.

WHERE SHOULD PREVENTIVE WORK TAKE PLACE?

Preventive work should take place where contact is made, either in the surgery or at home. Regular home visiting certainly establishes good relationships, and the importance of good relationships between doctor and patient cannot be overemphasised but it is possible to practice prevention without visiting every patient at home regularly. At least one member of the primary care team, however, should have paid a visit to every home so that someone is aware of home conditions, and the home visit should be repeated if circumstances change—when the patient has been discharged after admission for her first stroke, for example.

In old age

WHO SHOULD PRACTISE PREVENTION?

Who should practise prevention depends largely on the workload of the health visitor and district nurse, but every member of the primary care team has a part to play—especially the practice manager because of the need for an organised approach to prevention in old age.

REFERENCES

[1] Wilcock GK, Gray JAM, Pritchard PMM. *Geriatric problems*. Oxford: Oxford University Press, 1982.
[2] Gray JAM, Wilcock GK, *Our elders*. Oxford: Oxford University Press, 1981.
[3] Stott N, Davis RH. The exceptional potential in each primary care consultation. *J R Coll Gen Pract* 1979;**29**:201–5.

Adults

C F DONOVAN

"Prevention is the key to healthier living and a higher quality of life for us all."[1]

Preventive medicine, or "anticipatory care," is relevant to any patient who is seen by any doctor. Doctors, however, have time to undertake only a few of the tasks that are open to them, so they are forced to choose where to spend their resources. To some it may seem that the general practitioner should spend time with the most vulnerable patients, and this tends to be the young and the old. But a moment's thought will show that the choice is not easy. Healthy adults are essential in the life of many vulnerable patients. Parents conceive and rear children, break or make marriages, and inflict emotional or physical injury on their offspring. Mothers decide whether or not to attend antenatal clinics and to smoke or drink during pregnancy. Many old people and those who are chronically sick depend on another adult to shop or clean or care for them. Adults create the wealth of our country on which our medical services depend. In short, adults have a strong claim on the limited time of the general practitioner, both in curative and preventive medicine.

MORTALITY AND MORBIDITY

The overwhelming tragedy of death makes anything that the doctor can do to prevent it important. The four most frequent causes of death in adults are cardiovascular disease, cancer, cerebrovascular accidents, and accidents. These can be reduced by anticipatory care. Death rates from ischaemic heart disease have since the 1960s come down in the United States.[2] The variation of mortality figures in different countries (table I) shows the scope for prevention.

TABLE I—*Percentage of persons aged 45 years who will not survive to 65 years, given the death rates of 1972*

Country	Men (%)	Women (%)
Sweden	19	11
England and Wales	27	14
Scotland	31	18

Reproduced with permission from *Prevention and health: everybody's business.*[1]

Chapters in this book on prevention on coronary heart disease, hypertension, smoking, cancer, and alcohol all touch on the areas

73

Adults

where general practitioners can help to modify these horrifying statistics. It is important for us general practitioners to try and take a smoking and alcohol history on our patients and a blood pressure reading once a year. Those who smoke should be advised to stop and given a pamphlet on giving up smoking and then should be followed up at a further consultation. Those who have a drink problem should be given time to discuss it and those who have hypertension treated.

More patients should have regular cervical smears taken[3] and more should be followed up for intermenstrual and rectal bleeding and abnormalities in pigmented naevi and breast lumps. But we general practitioners need to look beyond the mortality figures and see how much can be done in the surgery to prevent less overwhelming illnesses in adults. I have space to list only a few ways in which morbidity figures might be altered by the general practitioner. The reader may add others.

Immunisation—The simplest effective preventive activity in the surgery is probably immunisation. Figures show that 13% to 20% of potentially fertile women are still without antibodies to rubella.[4] There were 1000 terminations of pregnancy on the grounds of damaged fetuses in 1969, and many children are born with damaged hearing as a result of rubella.[5] [6] General practitioners could do much to identify mothers at risk and immunise them. Many patients are still not protected against polio—a condition that is common in some countries of the world and can be imported and cripple many of the adults on our lists who are not yet immunised.[7]

Antenatal clinics—Adults could be encouraged by general practitioners to attend earlier and more regularly at antenatal clinics and well baby clinics.

Low back pain—Low back pain is said to cause the loss of 11·5m working days to industry (£220m in lost output).[8] Much could be done to inform adults on the proper ways of lifting, bending, sitting, and working, so as to protect their backs from injury.

Bowel disease—Bowel disease and constipation may be reduced by changing our diets. Patients should be informed of the benefits of roughage and low fat diets (see figure).

Iatrogenic disease—Above all, general practitioners should be specially concerned about those illnesses caused by medical care. General practitioners can do much to prevent unnecessary hospitalisation, investigation, surgery, and medication.

In addition, there is a great potential for providing preventive care in adults for the family doctor who is interested in the emotional needs of his patients. One marriage in four is now said to end in divorce. Self poisoning accounts for 15% of acute hospital admissions.[9] Forty four per cent of all known conceptions to married women with two or more

74

children are regretted, and terminations are still running high, even in middle aged women (table II)—and this despite widespread contraceptive services provided by general practitioners and family planning clinics. "By listening and being open" general practitioners can help some patients to first reveal and then face up to personal or psychosexual problems, as well as to some of the difficulties that arise in the middle years. The recent publication on prevention in psychiatric disorders by the Royal College of General Practitioners[10] shows how stress at times of "life changes" may be helped by the general practitioner anticipating this and discussing it with patients. Such changes include the loss of job/retirement; pregnancy; childbirth; bereavement; and the effects of a major operation.

The evidence shows that we general practitioners prefer to prescribe rather than talk to our patients. Ann Cartwright concluded in *General Practice Revisited*[11]: "In 1977 and 1964, two thirds of the

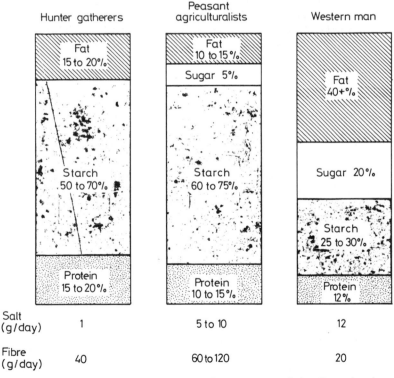

Contrasts in diet composition, comparing hunter-gatherers, peasant argriculturalists, and modern western man.

Adults

patients came away from the general practitioner's surgery with a prescription. . . . By 1977 the cost of drugs was more than one and a half times the cost of general medical services. . . . As a society we pay less for the advice, listening, and explaining, and the support that general practitioners give their patients than for the pharmaceutical products which they prescribe."

TABLE II—*Abortions in residents of England and Wales, 1976 to 1978*

Age (years)	1976	1977	1978
40 to 44	4520	4638	4918
45 to 49	463	511	482
50+	20	18	10
Total	5003	5167	5410

OTHER PEOPLE'S PRIORITIES

General practitioners may be helped in deciding their priorities with their primary care team by looking at those of others. The Department of Health and Social Security has three priorities: the reduction of cigarette smoking, alcohol abuse, and risk factors for ischaemic heart disease. The Royal College of General Practitioners in *Health and Prevention in Primary Care*[12] states: "In our opinion the most important opportunity for preventive care is at present:
—family planning;
—antenatal care;
—immunisation;
—fostering the bonds between mother and child;
—discouraging smoking;
—detection and management of raised blood pressure;
—helping the bereaved."
Prevention in all these areas requires that the general practitioner works with adults.

CAN THIS BE DONE BY THE GENERAL PRACTITIONER?

Many general practitioners are already overworked responding to the demands and wants of those who present themselves at the surgery. These demands are likely to increase as the education and expectations of patients grow, as surgeons and physicians discharge patients more rapidly from hospital, and as the proportion of elderly people increases. Every practising general practitioner knows that because of lack of time effective preventive work as described in this article cannot be achieved now. What general practitioners can do is plan for the future and make a start somewhere, perhaps remembering prevention in the consultation and also attempting to increase

76

their resources by getting extra support from other adults—for example, the self caring and responsibility of the patients themselves; other health professionals who work with the general practitioner, such as health visitors, district nurse, and midwife; members of patients' families; self care and voluntary agencies; and adults who decide on health policies.

When general practitioners feel the responsibility of preventive medicine weighing heavily on their shoulders they might remember that each adult ultimately carries the responsibility for his own and his family's health, and that each of the groups above carries a responsibility equal to that of the general practitioner for insuring that in the years ahead preventive medicine becomes a reality in our society.

FIRST PRIORITY

There is one adult who's health should, but often does not, take priority in the general practitioner's concern: the general practitioner's own health, if undermined, will have an effect on his practice and his family. Even minor physical and emotional upsets can play havoc with the running of the surgery and consultations. The Registrar General's figures for 1978 show that in Britain there are three conditions from which doctors are more likely to die than the general population. These and their respective standardised mortality ratios are suicide 335%, cirrhosis—that is, alcoholism—311%, and accidents 180%.[13] Two of these conditions have a psychological origin, and if combined with the fact that doctors have more marital problems than the rest of the population, indicates that the doctors' and their families' mental as well as physical health should be our concern.[14]

Yet how many general practitioners who practise preventive care include themselves? Apart from the medical profession's success with cigarette smoking (about one in five doctors in Britain still smoke) and the general practitioners who have attempted to study their emotional response to difficult patients by joining a Balint group, our profession's record is poor (table III).

TABLE III—*Items general practitioners might consider when thinking of their own health*

Registering with a general practitioner outside the practice
Having blood pressure checked once a year
Taking regular holidays
Having a minimum of exercise and a minimum of time with our families
Stopping smoking, reducing alcohol intake, and monitoring emotional responses to the frustrations and pressures of work and life
Preparing for retirement

CONCLUSION

Prevention added to curative medicine is the key to a higher quality

Adults

of life for many people. It is through adults that changes in attitudes will be brought about. Given the resources, there is much that general practitioners working with their adult patients can do to promote health and to prevent unnecessary physical and emotional illness. To achieve widespread improvement it is necessary to include social change. For it is in housing, employment, civil strife, pollution, and wars that many of the seeds of much ill health are sewn. The general practitioner has an obligation, both as an individual and through his professional bodies, to help to change the attitudes of adults in positions of power, so as to bring about for the next generation a society in which the priorities of health are given equal status with those of wealth.

The figure is reproduced with permission from an article by Mr Denis Burkitt, *Update* 1982;**24**:38. Table II is reproduced with permission from an article by Barbara Law, *Update* 15 April 1981.

REFERENCES

[1] Department of Health and Social Security. *Prevention and health: everybody's business.* London: HMSO, 1976.
[2] Stallones RA. The rise and fall of ischaemic heart disease. *Sci Am* 1980;**243**,No 5:43–9.
[3] Anonymous. Cervical cancer—the challenge to general practice. *J R Coll Gen Pract* 1982;**32**:69–72.
[4] Black NA. Provision of rubella immunisation in general practitioner family planning services. *J R Coll Gen Pract* 1981;**31**:593–5.
[5] Peckham CS, Martin JAM, Marshall WC, Dudgeon JA. Congenital rubella deafness: a preventable disease. *Lancet* 1979;i:258–61.
[6] Anonymous. 1500-2000 babies affected. *Br Med J* 1978;ii:1441.
[7] Strube G. Poliomyelitis—immunisation is still essential. *Modern Medicine* 1981;**26**:46–7.
[8] Working Group on Back Pain. *Report of the Secretary of State for Social Services.* London: HMSO, 1979.
[9] Anonymous. Suicide and deliberate self-injury. *J R Coll Gen Pract* 1981;**31**:580–1.
[10] *Prevention of psychiatric disorders in general practice.* London: Royal College of General Practitioners, 1981.
[11] Cartwright A, Anderson R. *General practice revisited: a second study of patients and their doctors.* London: Tavistock Publications, 1981.
[12] *Health and prevention in primary care.* London: Royal College of General Practitioners, 1981.
[13] Murray RM. Health of doctors; a review. *J R Coll Physicians London* 1978:**12**:403–15.
[14] Pereira Gray J. The doctor's family: some problems and solutions. *J R Coll Gen Pract* 1982;**32**:75–9.

Adolescents

ALEXANDER D G GUNN

Adolescence is an imprecisely defined time of life. It is presumably postpubertal and preadulthood, but chronologically both of these landmarks in human development vary with social, genetic, nutritional, and ethnic deviations from any arbitrarily chosen norm. Dependent on constant social change, however, it seems that in the developed world adolescence may extend from the age of 15 to 25. As an age group—just under 25% of the population in Europe and North America, but 50% of the population elsewhere—they provide the highest incidence of accidents, abortion, venereal disease, crime, drug addiction, and drunkenness, yet remain in strictly medical terms the apparently healthiest proportion of the whole population. The contrast of the high incidence of social ill health and maladjustment with the relative freedom from disease makes adolescents relatively rare consulters of general practitioners. The opportunity, therefore, for practising preventive medicine—particularly when one of the other characteristics of this age group is a high social and geographical mobility—is infrequent once they have left school or home. Nevertheless, effective prevention for the adolescent may be defined as being in two areas: the practical and the hopeful.

PRACTICAL PREVENTION

The need for immunisation and contraception provides the two most frequent opportunities for practising prevention that the general practitioner has with adolescent patients. Unfortunately, in neither case does the delivery seem to meet the demand. About 10% of young women enter their childbearing years unprotected against rubella, and about 11% of pregnancies are not wanted, which is increasing the demand for abortion each year. With regard to tetanus immunisation, school leavers are found in increasing numbers to require a booster, if not a full course, and every year universities and colleges find that more and more 18 to 19 year olds are insufficiently protected against poliomyelitis. With the absence of any requirement for routine medical surveillance after leaving school (and it is sparse enough at school) the general practitioner's contact with the adolescent depends almost invariably on illness occurring. In the days of age and sex registers and computerised records, however, it behoves the general practitioner to maintain an accurate record of the immune status of his adolescent patients and update it continually—not leaving it to casualty departments or antenatal clinics to define the person's need for tetanus or rubella protection. Similarly, with the greater frequency of foreign

Adolescents

travel—so often undertaken by the adolescent—providing separate immunisation clinics in the group practice to administer the polio, cholera, tetanus, typhoid, or gammaglobulin protection as well as the prescription for anti-malarial preparations is essential for effective prevention of tropical disease.

Contraception is sought seemingly more often by the adolescent female from the local clinic than from the family doctor—a recognition of the embarrassment in declaring publicly a private commitment to sexual activity. Nevertheless, many young people find the requirements of an internal examination and cervical cytology distinctly unacceptable and prefer to "chance it" at first, rather than approach their sexual adventures appropriately protected. By linking the provision of contraception with illness the medical profession may have contributed to the failure of its total acceptability. Every attempt should be made to overcome this. It is necessary to provide appropriate leaflets in the waiting room and well advertised clinics for check ups that are seen and known to be separate from normal surgery attendance for oral contraception prescriptions. Similarly, the "signal" symptoms of disorder from cystitis to vaginitis, or balanitis to warts in young men, should initiate a discussion of effective contraception. Recommending the use of sheaths to those with transmissible genital disorders until their treatment is effective would also go far to reduce the frequency of non-specific urethritis, monilia, trichomonas, and warts that seems to increase every year.

Injury on the sportsfield or at play, work, or on the roads is the next most frequent cause of contact with the general practitioner, and the need for the general practitioner to have access to facilities for physiotherapy is paramount. Rehabilitation of the active sportsman or woman is rewarding because of their enthusiasm to get better, and the development of keep fit and exercise classes as an adjunct to the service is distinctly lacking in the National Health Service. As a result separate—and extremely popular—sports injury clinics have developed in certain areas. Skills acquired from courses given by the British Association of Sports Medicine are rightly in high demand. Tuition in avoiding further injury and the proper way to keep physically fit is well repaid when offered to the earnest adolescent. If it cannot be done by access to specialised facilities then appropriate personal instructions and leaflets on exercises are necessary.

Skin disorders cause the next most frequent series of consultations, with acne, tinea in its various forms and sites of attack, verruccae, warts, dandruff, pediculosis, and scabies being the order of frequency. At each of these consultations verbal (and ideally, appropriately written) instruction and education about hygiene, washing, cosmetics, diet, and personal care are essential. Too often it is left to the commercial advertisement to instruct, not the doctor.

Measuring haemoglobin and blood count frequently is rewarded by the detection of ever present but insidious iron deficiency anaemia, from which one in 10 (both male and female) adolescents suffer, often undiagnosed until rejected by the Blood Transfusion Service. Growth, diet, injury, and menstruation are responsible.

HOPEFUL PREVENTION

The hopeful area for prevention in adolescence is the influence of the physician on the young person at each consultation. Obesity, smoking, alcohol consumption, and a misplaced reliance on some pharmacological preparation to solve a personal problem all fall into this area. Health education is much less effective by poster, leaflet, or advertisement than it is at the doctor's consultation, for the patient is at that time receptive to and anxious for advice. Height and weight charts can be distributed, a firm attitude to the use of tranquillisers and hypnotics shown, and a discussion of the individual's social life-style initiated—so that the doctor can learn too. The adolescent is naturally curious and requires clear sensible advice—not a sermon—for the myths of teenage culture to be laid.

SUMMARY

(1) Give effective and up to date immunisation.

(2) Provide contraception separated from the clinical routine of examination.

(3) Encourage the use of sheaths in all appropriate circumstances.

(4) Provide access to physiotherapy and instruction in physical fitness routines.

(5) Provide appropriate verbal and written information on personal hygiene and nutrition.

(6) Always offer advice, tempered with educational instruction.

Children aged 5 to 15

C F DONOVAN

During the years 5 to 15 many things happen to our patients. They move from home to school. They grow physically, emotionally, and sexually. Their attitudes are formed, and the skills of socialising, learning, and carrying responsibility are acquired. During this process some of our patients have to cope with handicaps and difficult emotional and physical environments. In this article I discuss a few of the areas in which general practitioners who "think prevention" can help these patients.

CLINICAL CARE (SECONDARY PREVENTION)

It is a mistake to think of prevention as separate from good clinical care (tables I and II). Nowhere is prevention more important than in recognising rare but serious conditions early. The case of meningitis, torsion of the testicle, malignant melanoma, or leukaemia that one sees only once in several years is still sometimes diagnosed late, with serious consequences. Less traumatic conditions that the general practitioner sees more often can, if not diagnosed early, also lead to unnecessary problems—for example, glue ear, appendicitis, scoliosis, and urinary reflux. Good clinical care and prevention also overlap when the general practitioner makes an effort to limit the medication, investigation, or hospitalisation of his young patient. Constantly questioning the need to prescribe drugs such as antibiotics, steroid creams, tranquillisers, or even cough linctuses, not only prevents iatrogenic illness but also prevents the breeding of attitudes in future adults that simple self limiting conditions require a doctor's consultation and prescription. Prevention in general practice also includes occasional curbing of enthusiasm for that extra investigation or even questionable operation, such as tonsillectomy.

CONTINUING MEDICAL CONDITIONS (TERTIARY PREVENTION)

The periodic supervision of the treatment of patients with chronic medical conditions by the general practitioner and the primary care team can prevent complications. Keeping the morbidity and age-sex registers up to date enables the team to identify and review school-children with diabetes, epilepsy, asthma, or fibrocystic disease and also those with physical and emotional handicaps or those in a one parent family. Preventing complications in these conditions may be achieved if good communications are built up and maintained with paediatric departments, the school medical service, and, above all, parents of the children concerned.

82

PRIMARY PREVENTION

In this book on prevention in general practice many subjects are discussed that are relevant to this age group, but some have special importance.

TABLE I—*Paediatric workload in general practice: percentage of patients and annual number of doctor contacts*

Age group (years)	No of consultations per year			
	0	1–5	6–10	10+
0–4	13·2	65·0	14·7	7·1
5–14	17·9	64·5	11·2	6·4

TABLE II—*Childhood illness in general practice. (Source: Office of Population Censuses and Surveys, 1974)*

Diagnosis	Episodes in a year (per 1000 population) Age (years)	
	0–4	5–14
Diseases of respiratory system	1009	521
Acute nasopharyngitis	470	152
Acute pharyngitis and tonsilitis	213	186
Acute bronchitis and bronchiolitis	185	73
Catarrh	48	22
Symptoms and ill defined conditions	343	168
Cough	113	49
Acute vomiting or diarrhoea or both	112	31
Infective and parasitic diseases	209	160
Measles, rubella, chickenpox, whooping cough	84	51
Intestinal infectious diseases	63	17
Viral warts	5	42
Diseases of nervous system and sense organs	312	161
Acute otitis media	186	83
Conjunctivitis and ophthalmia	70	19
Diseases of skin and subcutaneous tissues	214	150
Eczema and dermatitis	100	30
Infective conditions	55	60
Accidents, poisonings, and violence	92	113
Lacerations, abrasions, and superficial injuries	49	58
Sprains	10	28
All episodes	2873	1505

Immunisation

Ten to 20% of schoolgirls miss their school rubella immunisation.[1][2] It is theoretically possible for general practitioners to identify the patients who remain at risk and offer a back up service to that of the school medical service. Polio immunisation is especially important in older children who are going abroad, as is giving gammaglobulin to those who may be going to places where hepatitis is rife.

Children aged 5 to 15

Accidents

Accidents are the largest single cause of death in this age group (table III). Road accidents are the main cause, followed by accidents in the home; but drowning, suffocation, and poisoning must not be forgotten. Nearly 80% of children aged 5 to 9 who are killed or seriously injured in road accidents are pedestrians.[3] General practitioners and health visitors can do much to encourage families to become aware of the risks to their children and to consider reducing hazards in the home and the car, as well as seeing that their young children are well versed in road drill.

TABLE III—*Deaths from accidents, violences and poisoning (England and Wales 1976) (Source: Office of Population Censuses and Surveys, 1978)*

	Sex	Deaths by age group (years)			
		0–4	5–9	10–19	Total
All deaths due to accidents, poisoning, or violence	M	407	259	247	913
	F	241	135	112	488
Motor vehicle transport accidents	M	89	138	116	343
	F	48	73	49	170
Drowning	M	38	39	26	103
	F	17	13	7	37
Inhalation and ingestion of food	M	88	3	7	98
	F	34	1	1	36
Falls	M	31	18	21	70
	F	14	7	4	25
Accidental mechanical suffocation	M	23	3	24	50
	F	25	1	1	27
Homicide	M	35	1	3	39
	F	27	10	9	46
Poisoning	M	11	5	4	20
	F	6	3	4	13

Contraception

Two girls a day aged 15 or under now have therapeutic abortions in England, in addition to the unwanted illegitimate pregnancies that go to term. A quarter of all abortions performed in England and Wales since 1978 were performed on girls aged 15 to 19.[4] By developing a relationship with young patients general practitioners and health visitors may find an opportunity to raise the subject of sexuality and contraception at an appropriate time. General practitioners should inform young patients that contraceptive services can be provided without an internal examination. Care must be taken in discussing contraception with the under 15 year olds not to undermine parental responsibility. Some general practitioners prefer to discuss this with parents and encourage them to raise the subject with their children.

Nutrition

Improving the nutrition in this age group is fundamental to health, as it is to the care of their teeth. But there is a danger that the discussion of this subject may encourage the advertiser's false message that "thinness" and not "good nutrition" is what is desired. The mention of food or of obesity by the general practitioner must be done with care so as not to add to the growing incidence of eating problems, especially bulimia and anorexia.

Smoking, alcohol, and drug abuse

Smoking starts early. Bewley[5] showed in 1973 that in the final year in primary school 6·9% of boys and 2·6% of girls were regular smokers in Derbyshire. Attitudes to alcohol, glue sniffing, and experimentation with drugs are also formed early. Here the crucial influences on attitudes in developing children must be the family, the school, the media, and society at large. If general practitioners raise the subject of smoking or alcohol abuse with parents, especially within the hearing of the children, they may be able to counter some of these influences. Some general practitioners go further and give talks in schools, youth clubs, or on television. Others feel that as a profession we should bring more pressure on the media and other influences in society, including the soft approach of the government to the sponsoring of sports by tobacco industries.

Emotional, behavioural, and learning problems

There is a high incidence of emotional, behavioural, and learning problems during the years 5 to 15. Every general practitioner can recount his experience of parasuicides, anorexics, drug abuse, truanting, learning problems, and abnormal psychological and even criminal behaviour in the children on his list. It is a sad fact that we in general practice can do little to buffer our young patients from the influences of advertising, social change, and disintegrating marriages.

England now has the highest divorce rate in the EEC. "Currently one in four marriages is likely to end in divorce. Some 60% will involve dependent children . . . between one in five and one in six children born today may witness their parents' divorce before they reach 16."[6] Many children return to an empty home after school because their mother is out at work. One in seven children are now brought up in a one parent family. Many children suffer overprotective parents or parents who themselves are depressed and unable to give them the warmth they need. Far too many children suffer from inadequate housing and poor play facilities.

CAN THE GENERAL PRACTITIONER DO ANYTHING TO PREVENT SOME OF THESE PROBLEMS?

Here are a few suggestions, largely based on *Prevention of*

Children aged 5 to 15

Psychiatric Disorders in General Practice, published by the Royal College of General Practitioners.

—Attempt to identify "overprotective" mothers, and avoid encouraging children of these parents to be kept off school unnecessarily after illness.

—Emphasise to overprotective parents what their child can do on its own.

—Encourage as much as you can any form of support for children whose parents are unable to provide warmth, and make an extra effort to avoid hospitalising these children.

—Pay more attention over the long term to the children on the list who are in care and may be experiencing a rapid turnover in adults looking after them, and encourage social workers to have them fostered.

—Identify early and get remedial teaching for children who have learning difficulties or communication problems.

—Identify families where the parents have psychological or sexual difficulties and see if they can face these problems and accept help before it leads to breakdown of the marriage.

—Try to prevent children from being used by their parents as pawns when marriages do break down, by pleading the children's case.

CAN BUSY GENERAL PRACTITIONERS DO THESE THINGS?

Lists of desirable things that primary care teams can do for any age group are easy to compile. Those who work in general practice know how difficult it is to implement them. What children on our list need is that we do more than just read about prevention. In deciding if any of these suggestions could be implemented the reader might find the following of some help:

—It seems that much of the general practitioner's time is taken up in advising parents on simple self limiting conditions, such as colds, diarrhoea and vomiting, constipation, sprains, dandruff, etc, so that little time is left to deal with children's real needs in the field of prevention. Yet each consultation is an educational opportunity, one that can be extended by written material. The refusal of the doctor to prescribe for a cold, the advice to go to a chemist to buy something for dandruff or to advise on a high roughage diet for constipation are educational in themselves—so is handing out a pamphlet, such as *Minor Illness,* produced by the Health Education Council, which has been shown to increase parents' knowledge and reduce the number of surgery consultations.

—Picking out the preventive needs of one member of the family in the age group 5 to 15 is liable to give a false picture. The needs of a child are often the needs of the whole family. Preventing the father having a coronary or mother slipping into a depressive breakdown, or helping both parents to cope with a bad patch in their marriage, or with granny, may help our young patients more than any preventive measure mentioned above.

—General practitioners who "think prevention" should heed the warnings of Illich and not undermine but enhance the self coping powers of families so that they can carry their own responsibility for preventing sickness and promoting the health and development of all the members of their family.

A NEW SUGGESTION

The working party that wrote the Royal College of General Practitioner's document *Healthier Children—Thinking Prevention*,[7] suggests that general practitioners should put aside time for a special surgery to which those aged between 12 and 13—identified through the age-sex register—could be invited. In such a session for older children, run on the lines of the well baby clinic, general practitioners could show their interest in the development of these children and provide an opportunity to discuss problems that the patients might have found difficult to present at a consultation. The general practitioner could also do the following during these sessions: check height and weight; check for scoliosis; check for rubella status of girls; check for immunisation status of boys and girls; discuss attitudes to smoking, alcohol, or drugs; discuss academic progress; if appropriate,

TABLE IV—*Checklist for adolescents*

	Problems/abnormalities
History	
Establish relationship with patient	
Home relationships	
School relationships and progress	
Any other problems	
Physical examination	
Record weight and height	
Scoliosis	
Review	
Check immunisation status	
Girls: note rubella and rhesus status	
Teaching topics	
Anti smoking leaflet and advice	
Discuss puberty	
Sexual-contraceptive information as appropriate	
Discuss accidents and prevention	
Problems, plans, referral	

Adapted from Eggertsen SC, Schneeweiss R, and Bergmann JJ. An updated protocol for pediatric health screening. *J Fam Pract* 1980;**10**:No 1,25–37. Published by Appleton-Century Crofts.

raise the subject of contraception and attitudes to sexuality and sex problems that may be present; mention the general practitioner service available to his patient, and how the relationship with his general practitioner will change when he is 16 (table IV).

CONCLUSIONS

Time does not wait for the developing child. Since the Court report was published, a generation of children has grown seven years older without any appreciable changes being made in the child care services which, many agree, are in need of improvement. Collectively, general practitioners, through the Royal College of General Practitioners, have made a new attempt to rekindle the will of those concerned to implement these long called for changes, with special emphasis on prevention, by publishing *Healthier Children—Thinking Prevention*. For the sake of all future children it is vital that general practitioners, civil servants, politicians, and parents do not let the suggestions in this report go the way of those that have preceded it. In the meantime, this chapter has listed some ways in which general practitioners can begin to provide a better preventive service for those in the age group 5 to 15 years.

Tables I, II, and III are reproduced from *Child Health in the Community*, 2nd ed, 1980, R G Mitchell, editor, with the permission of Churchill Livingstone. Table IV is reproduced from *Healthier Children—Thinking Prevention*, with the permission of the Royal College of General Practitioners.

REFERENCES

[1] Jones SAM. Health education to improve rubella immunisation in schools. *Br Med J* 1980;**281**:649–50.
[2] Gilmore D, Robinson ET, Gilmour WH, Urquhart ED. Effect of rubella vaccination programme in schools on rubella immunity in a general practice population. *Br Med J* 1982;**284**:628–30.
[3] Valman HB. ABC of 1 to 7. Accidents. *Br Med J* 1982;**284**:578–80.
[4] Office of Population Censuses and Surveys. *Abortion statistics 1974–1978*. Series AB, 1–5. London: HMSO.
[5] Bewley BR, Halil T, Snaith AH. Smoking by primary schoolchildren: prevalence and associated respiratory symptoms. *Br J Prev Soc Med* 1973;**27**:150–3.
[6] Rimmer L. *Families in focus*. London: Study Commission on the Family, 1981:36.
[7] *Healthier children—thinking prevention*. London: Royal College of General Practitioners, 1982.

The first five years of life

GRAHAM CURTIS-JENKINS

The rewards of prevention in childhood are unique because the benefits may last a lifetime. A general practitioner who runs a child health clinic in his practice that offers immunisation, nutritional guidance including accurate weighing, health education including developmental guidance, and routine surveillance examination at key ages has laid the foundations for an effective programme of prevention for children. Unless organisation and effective management are given priority, however, the medical inverse care law ensures that those who would benefit most from such a service are least likely to obtain it. It is not enough to say that a lot of children are immunised or that most children attend for routine surveillance examination. The job is not worth doing at all unless all the non-attenders are identified and every effort made to bring them and the services provided together.

It is not difficult for the general practitioner with his lists of patients to define his target population. The organisation required to identify correctly the target population, keep the lists up to date, and run a routine examination programme using it is not complicated. It is not the health visitor's job, and every general practitioner who wishes to be effective should employ staff to do this work. Ideally, a well chosen clinic secretary should be responsible for running the clinics, efficient bookkeeping, and deploying medical time, matching it to the needs of the child population; but, above all else, the clinic secretary must be responsible for maintaining a register of all preschool children in the practice. This needs cooperation from the rest of the practice team to ensure that information on all transfers in and removals out, as well as changes of address, is given to her so that the list is as accurate as possible. From this master list the routine surveillance examination programme is run. The secretary should also be responsible for identifying non-attenders, telling the health visitors and doctors (including the patient's own doctor if the practice maintains personal lists of patients for each partner) of the non-attendance, and then making the necessary arrangements for further appointments or a home visit to be made.

The health visitors with the practice midwife (when there is one) and the doctor who is responsible for the paediatric clinic service make up the rest of the preventive child care team. When the team works as one, with, for instance, minimal interference from nursing managers outside the practice, it usually becomes the most dynamic part of the practice. The health visitors greatly benefit from having a clinic secretary with the responsibilities I have mentioned. Their work becomes more satisfying and, when every preschool child in the practice has been identified, more effective.

WHO DOES WHAT?

Demarcation disputes about who does what usually can be ended when the team asks itself the question: Who does what best? An untrained, unskilled doctor who takes it on himself to carry out all the developmental medical surveillance, including routine vision and hearing tests, is courting disaster. The health visitors, with their special skills in developmental paediatrics, are certain to do the job better. When a doctor is sufficiently skilled, trained, and motivated, however, the health visitors should then be able to give up this routine work to concentrate on the far more important tasks of counselling, family casework, health education, and even moving out into the community to work with client groups in, for instance, health education and social support programmes.

In our practice health visitors have given up routine vision and hearing testing to trained doctors, who have incorporated this into the routine medical surveillance examination. Instead, their hearing testing skills are channelled into testing the hearing of all preschool children who have recently had middle ear infection: 75% of children referred to specialist agencies because of hearing loss are detected in this way and 25% in the routine clinic examination at key ages.

The team will not function without regular contact. Weekly meetings that should take priority over all other commitments are essential. Policy matters on subjects such as immunisation should be agreed and adhered to. A consensus on treatment strategies for night waking, infant colic, and other common problems should be established. Every member of the team is diminished in the eyes of a young mother who gets different advice from each of them on a simple problem.

Examinations at key ages are the backbone of the preventive care programme in our practice. Careful timing ensures that all the examinations by appointment and all the mothers who come to the two paediatric clinics in the week who want to see a doctor about their children can be fitted in—one service without the other only creates problems and drives mothers away to obtain help and advice elsewhere.

A dynamic programme such as I have described often stimulates patients to run self help groups. These need supporting and encouraging. In our pratice the atopy self help group does sterling work and is strongly supported by the team. The cooperation of child minders in bringing minded children for routine clinic appointments is actively encouraged by the high esteem accorded to them by the team and by an enlightened local authority that allows them access to toy libraries.

The local child minder and play group association is also strong and sympathetic to our aims, so giving further possibilities of cooperation in the community and the free flow of information about children in that community.

PAEDIATRIC SURVEILLANCE

That more than 90% of children keep their first appointment at clinic for their routine surveillance examinations is a measure of our success—not in terms of organisation, but showing that we are offering a service that parents judge valuable and worth while. That, I believe, is the criterion of success on which all prevention programmes in general practice should be judged. The guidelines that govern our team's activities are these:

(1) The commitment to the philosophy of prevention is shared by all members of the team.

(2) Effective organisation is the key priority to ensure that no child is "lost" and that all are seen at regular, agreed intervals.

(3) Practice wide policy ensures that all sick children are seen on the same day that a request for a home visit or consultation is made. This is essential to free the clinics from the inappropriate task of treating sick children and physically separating the sick from the well during the clinic.

(4) Continuous audit of the team's effectiveness; immunisation rates; non-attendance rates; and disorder rates; regular spot checks of the team's target population register against the practice age-sex register to ensure that no child is lost, are carried out regularly and, when appropriate, acted on.

All members of the practice staff need to know what goes on in the child prevention programme and why. Caring for patients who are ill is their first priority. Asking the following questions regularly will help to ensure that your partners are making their contribution.

(1) Do all your patients know your practice arrangements?

(2) Do you know when one of your children is seen in an accident department or by a deputy—and do you find out why?

(3) Do you visit the local paediatric department?

(4) Do all children get regular surveillance?

(5) Do you explain to parents how to use the service you provide and make sure they understand?

If agreement is not sought early on the adequate provision of illness care the clinic service can become the quick way to see the doctor. In some community child health clinics 40% of all children seen suffer from acute illness. This is not really what preventive services are set up for!

Tasks for the primary health care team

	Practice secretary	Clinic nurse	Health visitor	General practitioner	Midwife
Conception and delivery			Preconceptual counselling; health education; mothercraft; relaxation classes; social support	Preconceptual counselling; check on family history, rubella immunity, etc; antenatal care shared with hospital	Meets mother on booking; shares antenatal care; makes home visit to assess home conditions; supervises home deliveries from delivery until the 14th day; supervises hospital deliveries from arrival home to the 14th day

DELIVERY: 95% hospital deliveries

	Practice secretary	Clinic nurse	Health visitor	General practitioner	Midwife
	Enters baby into yearbook and initiates child record from information given by health visitor		On 10th day after birth makes first visit to home; support visits made when required; mother and baby attend two clinics weekly to ensure regular contact; problems referred to own doctor or clinic doctor if convenient; children always referred to patient's own doctor	First visit when baby is home to introduce the mother to the baby's skills and examine the baby in front of mother; follow-up appointment, if necessary, arranged before 7 months of age	
7 months	Routine 7 month appointment sent; mother and child greeted on clinic day and shown into doctor; non-attenders noted and information given to general practitioner and health visitor; another appointment made; if fails to attend second appointment, health visitor delivers appointment personally to parent	When it is confirmed that baby is fit and there are no contraindications, triple vaccine and polio vaccinations started; full information given on side effects		7 month assessment, including vision and hearing checks; refer to appropriate agencies when necessary for specialist assessment	

Age	Immunisation	Appointment	Contact / advice	Assessment
8–9 months	Second immunisation			
12 months	Third triple vaccine and polio	Routine 12 month appointment sent and same arrangements as above		12 month assessment, as above
30 months	Measles immunisation; given at 18–24 months	Routine 30 month appointment sent and arrangements as above	Advice about play schools given (play groups in regular contact with health visitor about children with problems)	30 month assessment as above; check immunisation status for measles and advise having it
48 months	Preschool booster diphtheria and polio	Routine 48 month assessment as above	Continuing contact with children and parents, usually initiated by parents	48 month assessment, as above

COMMON TASKS

(1) Identify all children at risk from physical and emotional deprivation, sharing this information, and making decisions as quickly as possible about action

(2) Consensus approach to advice about commonly occurring problems, sleep problems, feeding problems, nappy rashes, and common variations in infant behaviour

(3) Regular weekly meetings to share information, discuss care strategies, and audit work of clinic. Social workers and speech therapists, orthoptists, students, and practice visitors are often present by invitation and contribute to the meetings in many positive ways.

Informal practice case conferences often prevent time consuming case conferences outside the practice and ease of communication facilitates decision making

INDIVIDUAL TASKS

(1) Updating of yearbook and age-sex register to ensure accuracy in identifying target populations
(2) Accurate recording of information

(1) Accurate recording of all immunisations on clinic record and patient's medical record envelope
(2) Regular updating and revising information on contraindications *as soon as* information is available

(1) Accurate recording of information about patient new to practice given by practice manager (and removals out) and sharing this information with clinic secretary
(2) Accurate note keeping

(1) Maintain all audit data and regular discussions of implications with rest of team
(2) Maintain developmental paediatric skills with updating of test procedures when necessary
(3) Accurate note keeping

(1) Maintain accuracy of birth data and regularly discuss implications with rest of team. Pass information when appropriate to the doctor in charge of the child surveillance programme or other member of the team about her concerns with mother and child

The health visitor and prevention

SHIRLEY GOODWIN

Prevention has been the raison d'etre of health visiting since the profession sprang into existence during the middle of the last century in response to the high infant morbidity and mortality rates in some northern cities. The official functions of the health visitor, as laid down by the statutory training body, include the prevention of mental, physical, and emotional ill health, the early detection of ill health, recognising and identifying need, health teaching, and providing care.[1] Preventive activity at each of Caplan's three levels of prevention[2] is clearly represented in these areas.

MOTHERS AND CHILDREN

The traditional focus for health visitors has been maternal and child health and, inevitably, preventive strategies with these groups have become more highly developed than with those groups who have come more lately to the attention of health visitors. Foremost of such strategies must surely be the routine home visiting of all families when a baby is expected or when there are children under 5 years of age. The opportunities for educating and giving advice to promote healthy living and for the early detection of illness or abnormality are obvious. But it is difficult to show the beneficial effect of such intervention since health visiting is a statutory service, parts of which may not be withdrawn to provide a control group against which to measure any effect. The introduction, however, of a regular home visiting programme (fortnightly from birth to 3 months, and then monthly until 6 months of age) to families with babies who are identified as having a statistically increased risk of "cot death" seems to have been associated with a reduction of six deaths per 10 000. R G Carpenter, in a paper on the evaluation of more health visiting for high risk children in Sheffield, said that the data suggest that this reduction in mortality (comparable to the number of lives saved by the treatment of paediatric cancers) could be attributed to the visits by health visitors.

Although health visitors are convinced of the value of routine visiting as a means of primary prevention, they sometimes have difficulty in persuading general practitioners that visiting healthy families is anything but a waste of time when there are sick patients to be followed up and supported and others with health related social problems with whom the health visitor (in the opinion of the doctor) could more usefully spend time. There is probably less disagreement about the value of developmental assessment as a preventive measure. In the practice where I worked until recently a weekly child health

94

clinic is held and children are seen by the health visitor and doctor at 6 weeks, 8 months, 2½ years, and 4 years of age. A medical examination is conducted at each check up, and the health visitor assesses the child's developmental progress. A screening test for hearing is carried out at 8 months at a separate session. The Royal College of General Practitioners child developmental record card is used to record observations and is kept in the medical notes. This arrangement is popular with parents, children, and health workers, not least for the continuity of care that such a system provides, and in my experience there are fewer failures to attend than when check ups are available only at the health authority clinic.

The need for routine medical examination to be an invariable part of developmental assessment has been challenged recently, and a new approach to screening is being adopted in which the health visitors conduct the assessments, using a structured screening tool. One example is the Denver Developmental Screening Test.[3] This test was developed in the United States but has been standardised[4] for use with British children, and has been used by health visitors in South Glamorgan since 1974. One important aspect of the test is that it contains a clear cut indication of when it is necessary to refer a child for more detailed medical assessment. I have been concerned in supervising student health visitors who are taught to use this test and have been particularly impressed with the thoroughness and practicality of the training programme, and how fast students gain confidence in the knowledge and skills relating to normal child development.

OTHERS

At the other end of the life cycle are the elderly people who are becoming a greater proportion of the general practitioner's list and the health visitor's case load. Health visitors are constantly aware that they are in contact with only a minority of the individuals over retirement age to whom they could be of some service in terms of prevention. Case finding with the help of the age-sex register is possible to do, but most health visitors have too great a case load to permit them to take on routine screening and visiting of all the elderly people that they, or their medical and nursing colleagues, would wish. This is unfortunate since the effectiveness of health visitors in this area has been long recognised,[5] and a recent study[6] has shown the positive effect of monthly visits by a health visitor on the health of elderly women, an effect that persists for at least six months after visits have ceased.

"The most important single cause of death in the United Kingdom is coronary heart disease," according to the Department of Health and Social Security,[7] and health visitors are very much aware of the part

95

The health visitor and prevention

they have to play in its prevention.[8] It begins with the advice that health visitors can give on infant feeding, and continues with the information about the harmful effects of smoking, and the benefits of exercise and relaxation, which may be incorporated into health education to individuals and groups, particularly of schoolchildren.

For some years I have been teaching groups of adults how to understand and cope with stress more effectively.[9] Patients who are being weaned off tranquillisers, or who have hypertension, migraine, phobic symptoms, and other stress related conditions are referred by their doctors or health visitors (though many are self referred) and attend a six week course of classes held in a general practitioner's surgery. The course covers subjects such as the ill effects of chronic drug use, alcohol, and tobacco, and other maladaptive coping mechanisms, but it emphasises positive ways of dealing with stress, including acquiring skills in muscular relaxation.

In a short article it is possible to refer only briefly to some areas of the preventive work that health visitors may do. I have omitted reference to much of their work, including the psychosocial support, which is given high priority, particularly in the work with young families. So I conclude by welcoming the recent recognition of the importance of prevention by the *other* key member of the primary health care team, as demonstrated by the publication of the reports of the Royal College of General Practitioners working party on prevention. At last there is a glimmer of hope among health visitors that their medical colleagues will begin to appreciate what they have been up to all these years!

REFERENCES

[1] *The function of the health visitor*. London: Council for the Education and Training of Health Visitors, 1967.
[2] Caplan G. *An approach to community mental health*. London: Tavistock Publications, 1961.
[3] Bryant GM. Use of the Denver developmental screening test by health visitors. *Health Visitor* 1980;**53**:2–5.
[4] Bryant GM, Davies KJ, Newcombe RG. Standardization of the Denver developmental screening test for Cardiff children. *Dev Med Child Neurol* 1979;**21**:353–64.
[5] Williamson J, Lowther CP, Gray S. Use of health visitors in preventive geriatrics. *Gerontologia Clinica* 1966;**8**:362–9.
[6] Luker K. Health visiting and the elderly. Occasional Paper No. 35. *Nursing Times* 1981;**77**:137–40.
[7] Department of Health and Social Security. *Avoiding heart attacks*. London: HMSO, 1981.
[8] O'Connor P. Prevention of coronary heart disease: is there a role for the health visitor? *Health Visitor* 1981;**54**:28–30.
[9] Goodwin S. Curbing the caveman in us. *Nursing Mirror* 1980;**150**,No 20:22–4.

Helping agencies

S A SMAIL

Although many programmes of preventive care can be put into effect using resources drawn solely from within the practice there are several other agencies whose help may be invaluable and who may contribute considerably to the success of preventive care.

LOCAL AGENCIES

Health authority services

Health authorities are concerned to ensure that there is an adequate level of preventive care in their areas, but an effective overall strategy in an area demands close cooperation between the community services provided by the authority and general practitioners. Health authorities often take responsibility for preventive care for certain groups of patients and may, for example, provide paediatric screening and immunisation clinics, family planning clinics, and cervical cytology clinics. Local practice and deployment of resources varies from one authority to another, but it is vital that there is good communication between those who are responsible for running the clinical services of the authority and local practitioners to avoid obvious gaps in the provision of preventive care or, on the other hand, unnecessary duplication of effort. Many community medicine specialists are now more sensitive to the potential for practising preventive care in the practice, since it is often more logical for activities such as immunisation, antenatal care, family planning, and cervical cytology to be provided by the practitioner. Community medicine specialists will be able to provide practitioners with advice about local epidemiology but also can often give specific advice about the practicalities of initiating a preventive programme, such as a screening programme for hypertension.

Carrying out a programme of preventive care in a practice will often require the services of district nurses, health visitors, and midwives, who are employed by the health authority. If a practice is planning a new initiative it is important to discuss the plans not only with the nursing staff but also with the nursing officer. There may be the need for resources, but often a need for further training as well. For example, if a treatment room sister is to help to run an immunisation clinic the health authority will need to be satisfied that the nurse is competent to undertake the additional tasks. Usually the specialist in community medicine will be able to advise if any problems arise.

Health education officer

Virtually all health authorities now have the services of at least one

97

Helping agencies

full time health education officer. He or she is responsible for coordinating health education services in the area or district and for providing advice and resources. Many health education officers have a background in nursing or health visiting and some in education. About a third of all health education officers have undertaken further training and hold the diploma in health education. Most are likely to hold this diploma in the future.

The health education officer can provide a most important service for practitioners. He routinely keeps health visitors fully informed about local health education plans and about new initiatives, but he will always be willing to provide direct advice to practitioners. He holds stocks of health education material, ranging from displays and posters to films and film strips suitable for different audiences. Most health education units stock the full range of pamphlets from the Health Education Council and Scottish Health Education Group and often many others as well, including material produced locally. Some units have the services of a graphic artist or audiovisual technician and will lend slide or film projectors.

Patient groups

Some practices have now set up patient participation groups, which can supply a valuable framework for a preventive campaign. The group itself may help to run the campaign and organise meetings of patients. In some areas community health councils have become interested in preventive care and run coordinated local campaigns. Some community health councils have taken a particular interest in tertiary prevention (managing established disease) by seeking out and publicising facilities for patients with chronic disease and disability. Other local groups may also be helpful. Mother and baby groups are often attended by the health visitor who may be able to influence the health beliefs of those attending the group, but subsequently individual members of the group may have a more general effect by disseminating ideas of preventive care in the community.

Although there has been a history of difficult relationships between some self help groups and the medical profession there is no doubt that many self help groups, such as branches of the Eczema Society, British Diabetic Association, British Epilepsy Association, Alcoholics Anonymous, or weight control groups, can be invaluable for many patients and can supplement the efforts of the practitioners in both secondary (early detection of disease) and tertiary prevention.

Local authority

The local authority must also be seen as an important resource. The education department is responsible for health education in schools and may welcome advice from local health visitors or doctors. Adult education programmes always include keep fit classes of various kinds. Patients can often be encouraged to take a little more exercise by joining a keep fit class, but other classes that aim at teaching new hobbies may also be valuable in helping patients to find new interests. Cooking classes may even help people to learn something about nutrition. Recently some local authorities have started to run classes that are based on the successful Health Education Council campaign "Look After Yourself" and include straightforward advice about diet and exercise.

Social services departments are responsible for running day centres for elderly people and in England and Wales employ occupational therapists—both of importance in tertiary prevention. They also have details of local self help groups.

Local media

Local newspapers often run features or series on aspects of preventive care. This may stimulate local interest that a practice can use to advantage. Editors always welcome ideas, and practitioners can often act as a resource themselves, either by writing for the newspaper or by providing material or ideas for a features writer. Local radio also has a considerable impact and many practitioners act as the popular local "radio doc." Although listeners may not remember a great deal of specific information given in radio chat programmes they do respond to the general tone of the programme. Producers always like doctors to discuss the latest headline catching miracle cure, but most radio doctors manage to temper their producers' enthusiasm and include regular preventive advice in their programmes.

NATIONAL AGENCIES

Central Information Service Foundation

An informal service is available free of charge to all practitioners in Britain and provides information and advice about all aspects of practice management. For example, practitioners may obtain advice about setting up an age-sex register, a recall register, or a morbidity register—any of which may be valuable in providing preventive care in the practice.

Health Education Council
Scottish Health Education Group

Both the Health Education Council and Scottish Health Education Group have similar functions as central coordinating bodies for health education activities. They publish leaflets and pamphlets, many of

Helping agencies

which are coordinated with national campaigns. Some are now specifically designed for general practice—for example, the Give Up Smoking kit. The Health Education Council also has a recources centre, which consists of a lending library and a collection of health education material including audiovisual aids and facilities for viewing. A bibliographic service is also available.

Voluntary organisations

Many charitable bodies produce educational material for patients with chronic disease—for example, the British Diabetic Association and the British Epilepsy Association produce excellent pamphlets. Some charities also produce leaflets and audiovisual aids that can be used when giving talks in the practice, in school, and in youth clubs, for instance. Many of these are of a general nature and not necessarily linked to specific disease. A comprehensive index of this material is published biannually,[1] and a full list of charitable organisations concerned in health care is available from the Family Welfare Association.

USEFUL ADDRESSES

BMA/BLAT Film Library
BMA House
Tavistock Square
London WC1H 9JP
Tel: 01-387-4499
Central Information Service Foundation
14 Princes Gate
London SW7 1PU
Tel: 01-581-3232
Family Planning Information Service
St Andrew's House
27-35 Mortimer Street
London W1N 7RJ
Tel: 01-636-7866
Family Welfare Association
(publishes *Charities Digest*)
501-503 Kingsland Road
Dalston
London E8 4AV
Tel: 01-254-6251
Health Education Council
78 New Oxford Street
(Resources Centre, 71-75 New Oxford Street)
London WC1A 1AH
Tel: 01-637-1881

Scottish Health Education Group
Woodburn House
Canaan Lane
Edinburgh EH10 4SG
Tel: 031-447-8044

REFERENCE
[1] Anonymous. *Health education index and guide to voluntary agencies.* London: B Edsall and Co, 1980.

How the Health Education Council can help

ALAN MARYON-DAVIS

Health education is the basic tool of prevention at all levels, from promoting healthy lifestyles to managing illness and rehabilitation. In primary care giving patients information and advice is a fundamental part of the job. Yet the practical difficulties of getting the salient facts across in the time available, so that they may be understood, remembered, and acted on, are often so daunting as to reduce the attempt to little more than lip service. But help is at hand through the local health education unit and from central organisations such as the Health Education Council.

HEALTH EDUCATION COUNCIL

The Health Education Council is a government funded but otherwise independent body, whose role is to promote and coordinate health education in England, Wales, and Northern Ireland. In Scotland the equivalent body is the Scottish Health Education Group. To the general public the most visible aspect of the Health Education Council's work is its mass media advertising campaigns, such as "Look After Yourself!" (diet, exercise, and smoking), "Superman" (children's smoking), and "Mother and Baby" (antenatal care). Less widely known is the extent to which health education has been promoted in schools by using specially developed packs of materials to facilitate teaching. But there are several ways in which the Health Education Council, working closely with the 400 or so health education officers throughout Britain who are employed by district health authorities, not the Health Education Council, can contribute more directly to health education in general practice.

PUBLICATIONS

The most immediate and practical support comes in the form of leaflets, booklets, and posters. There are 175 different items in the Health Education Council's publications catalogue, most of which are appropriate for use in general practice. All have a strong preventive bias and deal with subjects ranging from infant immunisation to self care for cystitis. Apart from posters and "pick up" leaflets for the waiting area, more and more booklets are designed specifically to support and extend the verbal advice given in the consultation. An example is the GUS kit (Give Up Smoking), which was developed jointly with Action on Smoking and Health. The package comprises a patient's booklet on how to give up smoking, a booklet with facts about smoking for the doctor, posters for the waiting room, and a note

How the Health Education Council can help

for the receptionist on how to use the kit. The patient booklet has the facsimile of a prescription form and the words "Give Up Smoking." By adding the patient's name and the practice stamp, the doctor can "personalise" the booklet so that the patient is more inclined to retain it and follow its advice. Another booklet for use by general practitioners is *Minor Illness: How to Treat It at Home*. This gives practical advice on self help for coughs, colds, sore throats, minor trauma, vomiting, and diarrhoea. It was written and evaluated by Morrell,[1] who found it had an important moderating effect on requests for consultations and home visits.

Like all Health Education Council publications, the GUS kit and *Minor Illness* may be obtained free of charge from district health education units, or, in case of difficulty, direct from the Health Education Council Supplies Section. The latest edition of the publications catalogue, including items in Welsh and Asian languages, may also be obtained from the same source.

USING LOCAL RADIO

There are nearly 60 local radio stations in Britain providing an important potential for health education. Although health experts, particularly general practitioners, are much in demand for interviews and phone ins, many opportunities are wasted through poor broadcasting technique. The Health Education Council, in conjunction with the BBC Local Radio Training Division, organises one day workshops in basic technique for beginners, offering practical advice in a real studio setting. Although intended primarily for doctors, the workshops are open to other health care personnel, tuition fees being met by the Health Education Council. Many of the doctors who have attended workshops are now regular broadcasters on local radio. Details are available from the author.

RESEARCH

The Health Education Council funds research into health education in general practice. For example, a major study undertaken by the Health Education Studies Unit has analysed over 2000 audio taped consultations to find ways of improving doctor-patient communications and using the many preventive opportunities that arise. Results will be published shortly. At the Welsh National School of Medicine the ways in which the lifestyle of working class mothers affects the attitude and actions they take to pursue health and avoid illness is being studied.

The Health Education Council is expanding its research funding in general practice and will consider projects on a large or small scale that have a substantial health educational element, especially if they relate

How the Health Education Council can help

to the Health Education Council' major programmes concerning heart disease, misuse of alcohol, or antenatal care.

TRAINING

One of the main aims of the Health Education Council is to promote the teaching of health education skills to health professionals. To this end the Health Education Council sponsors diploma courses, seminars, and workshops for nurses, health visitors, and doctors. More and more vocational training courses are incorporating sessions on health education in general practice, to which the local health education officer, or the Health Education Council itself, can contribute by providing speakers and teaching aids.

OTHER ACTIVITIES

On a broader front the Health Education Council can help less directly by contributing to the public's overall awareness of healthy lifestyles and how to cope with illness. By promoting health education in schools and by working closely with journalists and producers of radio and television programmes, the Health Education Council can help people to take on a greater responsibility for their health and to avoid illness. The Health Education Council has provided, literally, millions of booklets to back up various television series: most recently the three BBC series "Feeling Great," "Play it Safe," and "So You Want to Stop Smoking."

Important target groups for health education are those who shape our lives more than anybody else: politicians, planners, and managers in industry. In line with its politically independent status the Health Education Council attempts to put the view of health educators as a whole with regard to such issues as sports sponsorship by tobacco companies or nutritional labelling of foodstuffs.

FURTHER INFORMATION

The Health Education Council's regular newspaper *Health Education News* is sent free of charge to those who request it. Further information on any aspect mentioned in this article may be obtained by writing to the author at the address below:

> The Health Education Council
> 78 New Oxford Street
> London WC1A 1AH

> The Scottish Health Education Group
> Woodburn House, Canaan Lane
> Edinburgh EH10 4SG

REFERENCE

[1] Morrell DC, Avery AJ, Watkins CJ. Management of minor illness. *Br Med J* 1980;**280**:769–71.

Prevention: who needs it?

NICK BLACK, P M STRONG

We begin with definition and end with speculation, for our topic is the possible social consequences of a massive extension of preventive medicine at the clinical level–a topic of considerable importance yet on which there is little definite knowledge. There are, of course, two sorts of preventive medicine. "Direct prevention" is concerned with the intention, choice, will, and responsibility of the individual. By contrast, through the judicious use of structural regulations and incentives, "indirect prevention"—though it still requires the consent of the politically influential—may be achieved without the assent or perhaps even the knowledge of major sections of the population.

The great programme of preventive medicine initiated by the Victorians and currently attracting renewed support in community medicine,[1][2] has operated mostly, though not entirely, at the indirect level. The new preventive medicine has a different emphasis.[3][4] Fiscal and legislative measures are certainly part of it, but its most distinctive thrust is direct action at the individual. Since this is its novel aspect, and since it is here that general practitioners are now being urged to play a major part,[5] it is on this that we shall concentrate.

Any comment must necessarily be speculative. Nevertheless, since space is limited, things must be said without qualification. Where we say typically, we do not mean universally. Moreover, there are many general practitioners who do not fit our model of current practice. Even so, the consequences of adopting direct, systematic prevention may well apply to all.

PREVENTION AND THE GENERAL PRACTITIONER

We begin with a highly simplified model. At present the standard consultation looks very crudely something like this: curative and palliative medicine are practised, preventive medicine is avoided; the biological side is stressed, while the social is played down; the organic is preferred to the psychiatric, and the patient's or, indeed, the doctor's personal responsibility is glossed over.[6] Put another way, doctor and patient both conspire to cast disease firmly into the natural realm, the realms of the body and of pure chance. Moral matters, on the surface at least, are systematically avoided. How patients choose to live is entirely up to them. It is entirely their business, not their doctor's. Direct prevention, however, if pursued systematically would sweep all this away. This could result in the following consequences for medical practice.

Prevention: who needs it?

A focus on men

Women are significantly more dependent on medicine than men; they are the principal lay carers; they are more vulnerable to diagnosis in psychiatric rather than organic terms[7]; above all, if they are also young mothers they are the only important group in the population at whom systematic and direct preventive medicine has been aimed. Mothers are, of course, particularly receptive or vulnerable to this approach. Extending it to men seems a much tougher proposition, though so far this has not been put to the test. If it can be achieved a central part of the traditional male image will have gone. To help them in this doctors may appeal to women, thus reinforcing their traditional role.[8]

A re-emphasis on social class

The working classes have appreciably higher rates of mortality and morbidity,[9] their uptake of preventive services is lower, and their orientation to prevention in general is definitely less, particularly among the lower working class.[10] Yet, at the same time, studies of general practice consultations suggest that doctors, far from attempting to do more with their working class patients, actually offer them less medical information.[11] General practitioners now leave detailed modification of the lifestyle of the lower classes to others, such as health visitors. They will no longer be able to do so.

Changes in the relationship between the general practitioner and the patient

Direct prevention is likely to modify drastically the standard doctor-patient relationship. Two effects in particular stand out. Whatever their actual knowledge patients typically play dumb and doctors play wise. More crucially perhaps, doctors commonly invest their individual clinical opinion with the authority of agreed professional judgment.[6] They can do so because in both curative medicine and public health medical knowledge remains, by and large, the property of professionals. Any credible and long term concern of patients in prevention, however, may teach them the uncertainties as well as the certainties of medicine, about the diversity of professional opinion,[12 13] and about the continually changing nature of "scientific truth."

Medicine is also one of the polite professions. Policemen and prosecuting counsel are obliged to be systematically rude. Doctors, however, have no need of this so long as they conspire with their patients to naturalise all disease and cast it into the realm of chance and the organic. All this might well change with the onset of detailed and direct prevention. Medical work would become moral work, and

106

patients might insist on a much greater freedom to choose and change their practitioner. This pressure for greater choice would also be strengthened by any weakening of individual clinical authority.

Attempts to counteract some of these effects may lead some general practitioners to restrict themselves to their traditional organic and curative role and leave direct prevention to other health professionals. By carefully segregating themselves they may thus avoid any challenge to their individual authority, the necessity of being rude occasionally, and the danger of scaring away sick patients who they might cure. Direct prevention is also an extremely time consuming business. To be effective, current lay health beliefs and practices must be understood, something which few doctors and social scientists currently investigate.[10] [14] In addition, in such a sensitive moral area the successful reformer must often move slowly and delicately. Six minutes for consultations is hardly likely to prove long enough for many patients.

Finance and liberty

Direct prevention seems to give the possibility of an appreciable reduction of costs which are presently borne by the state and the individual. To the general public it offers a chance of less disease; to the radical middle class it embodies romantic ideals of self help[15]; to government it offers the possibility of reduced overall expenditure.[16] Yet direct prevention itself will have costs, and these too must be accounted for. The following questions need some consideration.

Will more preventive medicine reduce overall health costs, given both the power of the traditional health sector and the increasing salience of medicine that it may foster?

In the knowledge that some preventive strategies turn out to cost more[17] how much more are we prepared to pay?

What can be done to minimise the deleterious effects of direct prevention—guilt and anxiety on the part of the patient, victimisation on the part of the doctor?

Is the marked extension of the medical empire compatible with the liberty of the individual? Is that liberty any more compatible with indirect than direct prevention?

Having successfully taken control of people's bodies[18] should medicine now attempt the expropriation of their minds?

For a profession that has prized its own independent status so highly, does an interest in direct prevention represent a rather different valuation of the patient's independence?

All this can be put more dramatically by invoking one possible future scenario.

Prevention: who needs it?

The spectre of universal chronic status

Curative and palliative medicine is now marginal to the lives of most adults. It is salient only to elderly people, to children, to chronically sick people, and to medical personnel. The advent, however, of preventive medicine which is scientifically based, armed with detailed knowledge of the individual's biochemistry, genetic structure, and social situation, might render it central to everyone. In such a world all of us would have chronic disease status, all of us would live "the life of the diabetic" or be under great pressure to do so. In such a world the words of Goethe,[19] written close to the beginning of the scientific revolution, would finally have come true:

"... I think it is actually true that humanity will win eventually. However, I am afraid at the same time the world will be a huge hospital and one will be the humane nurse of the other."

Thanks to Linnie Price, Klim McPherson, and Bob Dingwall for their helpful comments, and to Pam Hughes for typing the result.

REFERENCES

1 Smith A. Doctors in need of a cure. *Times Higher Educational Supplement* 1981 Apr 3:8–9.
2 Report of a Study Group. *Rethinking community medicine: towards a renaissance in public health.* London: Unit for the Study of Health Policy, June 1979.
3 Department of Health and Social Security. *Prevention and health: everybody's business.* London: HMSO, 1976.
4 *Look after yourself.* London: Health Education Council, 1979.
5 *Health and prevention in primary care.* London: Royal College of General Practitioners, 1981.
6 Strong PM. *The ceremonial order of the clinic.* London: Routledge and Kegan Paul, 1979.
7 Armitage KJ, *et al.* Response of physicians to medical complaints in men and women. *JAMA* 1979;**241**:2186–7.
8 British United Provident Association. *The man in your life.* Health promotion leaflet.
9 Report of a research working group. *Inequalities in health.* London: DHSS, 1980.
10 Blaxter M, Paterson E. Attitudes to health and use of health services of two generations of women in social classes IV and V. *Report to DHSS/SSRC joint working party on transmitted deprivation.* 1980.
11 Pendleton D, Bochner S. The communication of medical information in general practice consultation and the function of patient's social class. *Soc Sci Med* 1980;**14a**, 660–73.
12 McMichael J. Fats and atheroma: an inquest. *Br Med J* 1979;i;173.
13 Mann JI. Fats and atheroma: a retrial. *Br Med J* 1979;i:732–4.
14 Helman CG. General practitioners as social anthropologists. *Br Med J* 1981;**282**:787–8.
15 Robinson D, Henry S. *Self-help and health.* Oxford: Martin Robertson, 1977.
16 Department of Health and Social Security. *Care in action.* London: HMSO, 1981.
17 Sinclair C. Costing the hazards of technology. *New Scientist* 1969;**44**:120.
18 Illich I. *Limits to medicine.* London: Marion Boyars, 1976.
19 von Goethe JW, cited by Fliedner T. In: *Priorities for the uses of resources in medicine.* Fogarty International Centre proceedings No 40. Washington DC: Department of Health, Education and Welfare, 1976:132.

Index

Index

Index

Index